Essential Psychiatry: A Handbook

N.B. Singh

DEDICATION

To Nature,

I dedicate this book to you, the source of all life. You are my inspiration, my teacher, and my friend.

Thank you for teaching me about the beauty of the world around me. Thank you for showing me the power of the natural world. Thank you for giving me a sense of peace and tranquillity.

I promise to do my part to protect you and your many wonders. I will teach my children about the importance of conservation and sustainability. I will work to make the world a better place for all living things.

Thank you for everything, Nature.

With love,

N.B Singh

Contents

Welcome to *Essential Psychiatry: A Handbook*. This book aims to be a comprehensive and accessible guide to the multifaceted world of psychiatry. Designed for students, practitioners, and researchers, this handbook navigates through the complexities of mental health with a focus on providing essential knowledge and practical insights.

Navigating Psychiatry

Understanding mental health is a journey that involves exploring the intricacies of the mind, the interplay of biological and environmental factors, and the dynamic nature of psychological well-being. *Essential Psychiatry* is crafted to be your compass in this intellectual terrain. It is not just a textbook but a companion, offering a blend of theoretical foundations and real-world applications.

Key Features

Comprehensive Coverage

This handbook covers a spectrum of topics, ranging from the fundamentals of psychiatric disorders and assessment techniques to advanced treatment modalities, cultural considerations, and emerging technologies. Each section is meticulously crafted to provide a balance between theoretical knowledge and practical applications.

Mathematical Integration

In a unique approach, we integrate mathematical formulas and equations throughout the book. This inclusion serves to enhance the precision and analytical understanding of psychiatric concepts. Whether you're interpreting research findings, evaluating treatment outcomes, or navigating the complexities of psychiatric assessments, the mathematical insights provided here aim to empower your understanding.

Interdisciplinary Insights

Recognizing that psychiatry exists at the intersection of various disciplines, this handbook incorporates insights from neuroscience, psychology, pharmacology, and more. The interdisciplinary approach ensures that readers gain a holistic understanding of mental health, preparing them for the collaborative nature of modern psychiatric practices.

Who Should Read This Book?

Essential Psychiatry is tailored for a diverse audience:

- **Students:** Whether you are a medical student, psychology major, or pursuing any mental health-related discipline, this handbook serves as a foundational guide for your academic journey.

- **Practitioners:** For psychiatrists, psychologists, therapists, and other mental health professionals, this book provides a valuable resource for staying updated on contemporary practices and refining your skills.

- **Researchers:** If you are engaged in psychiatric research, the integration of mathematical insights and comprehensive coverage will aid in designing studies, analyzing data, and interpreting findings.

How to Use This Handbook

Each chapter is structured to facilitate easy navigation. Key concepts are highlighted, case studies are presented for practical application, and mathematical formulations are seamlessly integrated to deepen your understanding. Whether you read it cover to cover or use it as a reference guide, *Essential Psychiatry* is designed to be an engaging and informative companion.

Let the Journey Begin

As you embark on this journey through the pages of *Essential Psychiatry: A Handbook*, we hope you find it intellectually stimulating, practically relevant, and a source of inspiration for your pursuits in the fascinating field of psychiatry.

Chapter 1

Introduction

1.1 Overview of Psychiatry

$$\text{Psychiatry} = \sum_{i=1}^{n} (\text{Mind} \times \text{Brain}) + \int_{t=0}^{\infty} \text{Therapy}(t)\, dt \qquad (1.1)$$

In this equation:

$$\text{Mind} = \text{Emotions} + \text{Thoughts} + \text{Behaviors}$$

$$\text{Brain} = \text{Neurotransmitters} + \text{Neural Networks} + \text{Genetic Factors}$$

$$\text{Therapy}(t) = \text{Psychotherapy} + \text{Medication} + \text{Supportive Interventions}$$

The equation captures the essence of psychiatry, emphasizing the interplay between the mind and the brain, influenced by various factors over time. The therapeutic interventions evolve dynamically, adapting to the needs of individuals.

Key Elements:

- Mind: Emotions, thoughts, and behaviors.

- Brain: Neurotransmitters, neural networks, and genetic factors.

- Therapy(t): Psychotherapy, medication, and supportive interventions over time (t).

1.2   Historical Perspectives

Ancient Wisdom Equation:

$$\text{Ancient Wisdom} = \frac{\text{Philosophy} + \text{Spirituality}}{\text{Time}}$$

The ancient perspectives on mental health were shaped by the delicate balance between philosophy and spirituality over time.

Middle Ages Transformation:

$$\text{Transformation} = \text{Alchemy} \times \text{Observation}$$

During the Middle Ages, the transformation in understanding mental states involved an alchemical blend of knowledge and careful observation.

Enlightenment Enlightenment:

$$\text{Enlightenment} = \sqrt{\text{Reason} + \text{Empiricism}}$$

The Age of Enlightenment brought a radical shift in psychiatric thinking, emphasizing the square root of reason and empiricism.

Industrial Revolution Equation:

$$\text{Industrial Revolution} = \text{Technology} + \text{Urbanization}$$

The Industrial Revolution accelerated changes in psychiatry, driven by advancements in technology and the shift toward urban living.

Modern Synthesis Formula:

$$\text{Modern Synthesis} = \text{Biology} + \text{Psychology} + \text{Sociology}$$

The modern era witnessed the synthesis of biological, psychological, and sociological perspectives in understanding mental health.

These symbolic equations represent key historical periods, acknowledging the multifaceted influences that have shaped the field of psychiatry.

1.3   Current Trends and Challenges

Trends Quotient:

$$\text{Trends Quotient} = \frac{\text{Technology} + \text{Interdisciplinarity}}{\text{Time}}$$

Current trends in psychiatry are propelled by the rapid integration of technology and the fostering of interdisciplinary collaborations over time.

Challenge Equation:

$$\text{Challenge} = \text{Stigma} \times \left(\frac{\text{Access Issues} + \text{Resource Gaps}}{\text{Awareness}} \right)$$

The challenges in modern psychiatry are compounded by the persistence of stigma, intertwined with issues of limited access and resource gaps relative to the level of awareness.

Innovation Formula:

$$\text{Innovation} = \text{Research} + \text{Adaptability} + \text{Patient-Centeredness}$$

Addressing current challenges requires continuous innovation, driven by research, adaptability to evolving needs, and a commitment to patient-centered care.

Resilience Index:

$$\text{Resilience Index} = \frac{\text{Community Support} + \text{Mental Health Literacy}}{\text{Adversity}}$$

Measuring the resilience of mental health systems involves evaluating the collective impact of community support and mental health literacy relative to adversity.

These symbolic equations offer a creative way to represent the dynamic interplay of trends and challenges in contemporary psychiatry.

1.4 Scope and Importance

Scope Function:

$$\text{Scope} = \text{Complexity} \times \left(\frac{\text{Mind} + \text{Brain}}{\text{Integration}} \right)$$

The scope of psychiatry is intricately linked to the complexity of understanding the mind and brain, emphasizing the importance of their integrated exploration.

Importance Index:

$$\text{Importance} = \frac{\text{Public Health Impact} + \text{Quality of Life Enhancement}}{\text{Stigma Reduction}}$$

The importance of psychiatry is measured by its impact on public health and the enhancement of quality of life, balanced against efforts to reduce stigma.

Holistic Equation:

$$\text{Holistic Approach} = \text{Biopsychosocial Model} \times \text{Cultural Sensitivity}$$

The holistic approach in psychiatry integrates the biopsychosocial model with cultural sensitivity, highlighting its significance in comprehensive mental health care.

Innovation Constant:

$$\text{Innovation} = \text{Research} + \text{Adaptability} + \text{Ethical Practice}$$

The ongoing importance of psychiatry relies on a constant commitment to innovation through research, adaptability to evolving needs, and ethical practice.

These symbolic equations offer a creative representation of the scope and importance of psychiatry, emphasizing the integration of various elements for a holistic understanding.

1.5   Ethics in Psychiatry

Ethical Framework:

$$\text{Ethics} = \frac{\text{Autonomy} + \text{Beneficence} + \text{Nonmaleficence} + \text{Justice}}{\text{Compassion}}$$

In psychiatry, ethical decisions are guided by the delicate balance of autonomy, beneficence, nonmaleficence, and justice, all underpinned by a foundation of compassion.

Trustworthiness Quotient:

$$\text{Trustworthiness} = \frac{\text{Transparency} + \text{Honesty}}{\text{Confidentiality Breach}}$$

Maintaining trust in psychiatric practice involves upholding transparency and honesty, guarded against any breach of confidentiality.

Therapeutic Alliance Constant:

$$\text{Therapeutic Alliance} = \text{Empathy} + \text{Respect} + \text{Cultural Competence}$$

The foundation of the therapeutic alliance in psychiatry is built upon a constant interplay of empathy, respect, and cultural competence.

Informed Consent Equation:

$$\text{Informed Consent} = \text{Information Clarity} \times \left(\frac{\text{Voluntariness}}{\text{Capacity}} \right)$$

The ethical principle of informed consent requires clear information, ensuring voluntariness while considering the capacity of individuals to make decisions.

These symbolic equations offer a creative way to represent the ethical considerations in psychiatry, emphasizing the delicate balance and dynamic interplay of various ethical principles.

1.6 Key Terminologies

Psychiatric Glossary Function:

$$\text{Psychiatry} = \text{Mind} + \text{Brain} + \text{Behavior} + \text{Emotion} + \text{Diagnosis} + \text{Treatment}$$

The core of psychiatry involves the interplay of the mind, brain, behavior, emotion, diagnosis, and treatment, forming the foundation of the psychiatric glossary.

Diagnostic Precision Equation:

$$\text{Diagnostic Precision} = \text{Sensitivity} + \text{Specificity} + \text{Positive Predictive Value} + \text{Negative Predictive Value}$$

Achieving diagnostic precision in psychiatry relies on the balance between sensitivity, specificity, positive predictive value, and negative predictive value.

Therapeutic Outcome Constant:

$$\text{Therapeutic Outcome} = \text{Patient Engagement} + \text{Adherence} + \text{Therapeutic Alliance}$$

Optimal therapeutic outcomes in psychiatry are influenced by a constant interplay of patient engagement, adherence, and the therapeutic alliance.

Neurotransmission Formula:

$$\text{Neurotransmission} = \text{Synthesis} + \text{Release} - \text{Reuptake}$$

Understanding key terminologies involves grasping the delicate balance of neurotransmission, encompassing synthesis, release, and reuptake processes.

These symbolic equations offer a creative way to represent key terminologies in psychiatry, emphasizing the dynamic and interconnected nature of psychiatric concepts.

Chapter 2

Psychiatric Disorders

2.1 Mood Disorders

Mood Equation:

$$\text{Mood} = \text{Emotion} + \text{Intensity} + \text{Duration}$$

Mood disorders involve a complex interplay of emotion, intensity, and duration, where disruptions in this equilibrium contribute to the manifestation of mood-related conditions.

Depression Spectrum:

$$\text{Depression} = \frac{\text{Biological Factors} + \text{Psychosocial Factors}}{\text{Resilience}}$$

The spectrum of depression is influenced by a combination of biological and psychosocial factors, moderated by an individual's resilience.

Mania Index:

$$\text{Mania} = \text{Elevated Mood} + \text{Increased Energy} + \text{Impulsivity}$$

Mania, a characteristic of bipolar disorders, is defined by elevated mood, increased energy levels, and impulsivity, creating a distinctive index for diagnosis.

Neurotransmitter Imbalance:

$$\text{Neurotransmitter Imbalance} = \text{Serotonin} - \text{Dopamine} + \text{Norepinephrine}$$

Mood disorders often involve a delicate imbalance in neurotransmitters, particularly alterations in serotonin, dopamine, and norepinephrine levels.

These symbolic equations offer a creative way to represent aspects of mood disorders, emphasizing the multifactorial nature of their development and manifestation.

2.2 Anxiety Disorders

Anxiety Formula:

$$\text{Anxiety} = \sqrt{\text{Worry} + \text{Fear} + \text{Uncertainty}}$$

Anxiety disorders involve the square root of worry, fear, and uncertainty, capturing the multi-dimensional nature of anxious experiences.

Panic Equation:

$$\text{Panic} = \text{Sudden Fear} \times \left(\frac{\text{Heart Rate}}{\text{Calmness}} \right)$$

Panic attacks manifest as sudden fear, intensifying with an accelerated heart rate relative to the baseline calmness level.

Phobia Ratio:

$$\text{Phobia} = \frac{\text{Specific Fear}}{\text{General Courage}}$$

Phobias arise from specific fears, expressed as a ratio relative to an individual's general courage.

Neurotransmitter Symphony:

$$\text{Neuro Symphony} = \text{GABA} + \text{Serotonin} - \text{Dopamine}$$

Anxiety disorders involve a neurotransmitter symphony, with GABA and serotonin playing calming notes, while dopamine introduces an element of arousal.

These symbolic equations aim to creatively capture the essence of anxiety disorders, making them more engaging and memorable.

2.3 Psychotic Disorders

Psychosis Equation:

$$\text{Psychosis} = \text{Reality Warping} + \text{Hallucinations} + \text{Delusions}$$

Psychotic disorders manifest as a combination of reality warping, hallucinations, and delusions, symbolized by the equation.

Schizophrenia Signature:

$$\text{Schizophrenia} = \frac{\text{Positive Symptoms} + \text{Negative Symptoms}}{\text{Cognitive Dissonance}}$$

Schizophrenia exhibits positive and negative symptoms, their ratio contributing to a cognitive dissonance characteristic of the disorder.

Reality-Distortion Molecule:

$$\text{Reality Distortion} = \text{Dopamine Overdrive} + \text{Glutamate Imbalance} - \text{Serotonin Dips}$$

Psychotic episodes involve a molecular dance with dopamine overdrive, glutamate imbalance, and serotonin dips leading to reality distortion.

Neurotransmitter Chaos:

$$\text{Neuro Chaos} = \text{Dopamine} \times \text{Glutamate} + \text{Serotonin}$$

Psychotic disorders disrupt the delicate neurotransmitter balance, creating chaos with the interplay of dopamine, glutamate, and serotonin.

These symbolic equations offer a creative way to represent psychotic disorders, emphasizing the complex interplay of symptoms and neurotransmitter dynamics.

2.4 Personality Disorders

Personality Equation:

$$\text{Personality} = \text{Traits} + \text{Patterns} + \text{Inflexibility}$$

Personality disorders emerge from a combination of enduring traits, maladaptive patterns, and inflexibility in behavior, symbolized by the equation.

Narcissism Coefficient:

$$\text{Narcissism} = \frac{\text{Self-Importance} + \text{Empathy Deficit}}{\text{Reality Check}}$$

Narcissistic personality disorder involves an elevated self-importance and an empathy deficit, forming a ratio relative to the ability for a reality check.

Borderline Rollercoaster:

$$\text{Borderline} = \text{Intense Emotions} + \text{Unstable Relationships} + \text{Identity Crisis}$$

Borderline personality disorder is like a rollercoaster ride, characterized by intense emotions, unstable relationships, and identity crises.

Cluster B Mix:

$$\text{Cluster B} = \text{Dramatic} + \text{Erratic} + \text{Impulsive}$$

Personality disorders in Cluster B (e.g., narcissistic, borderline) share traits of being dramatic, erratic, and impulsive.

These symbolic equations offer a creative way to represent personality disorders, emphasizing key components and traits associated with these conditions.

2.5 Neurodevelopmental Disorders

Neuro Development:

$$\text{Neuro Development} = \text{Genes} + \text{Environment} + \text{Neural Wiring}$$

Neurodevelopmental disorders arise from the interplay of genetic factors, environmental influences, and the intricate wiring of neural connections.

ADHD Formula:

$$\text{ADHD} = \frac{\text{Inattention} + \text{Hyperactivity} + \text{Impulsivity}}{\text{Focus}}$$

Attention-deficit/hyperactivity disorder (ADHD) involves a balance between inattention, hyperactivity, and impulsivity relative to one's ability to maintain focus.

Autism Spectrum Equation:

$$\text{Autism Spectrum} = \text{Social Challenges} + \text{Repetitive Behaviors} + \text{Communication Differences}$$

The autism spectrum encompasses challenges in social interaction, repetitive behaviors, and differences in communication skills.

Intellectual Dance:

$$\text{Intellectual Dance} = \text{IQ} \times \left(\frac{\text{Adaptive Functioning}}{\text{Challenges}} \right)$$

Intellectual disability involves a dance between IQ and adaptive functioning, modulated by the challenges an individual faces.

These symbolic equations offer a creative way to represent neurodevelopmental disorders, emphasizing the multifactorial nature and characteristics associated with these conditions.

2.6 Substance-Related and Addictive Disorders

Addiction Equation:

$$\text{Addiction} = \text{Substance Use} + \text{Craving} + \text{Tolerance} + \text{Withdrawal}$$

Addictive disorders involve a combination of substance use, intense cravings, tolerance development, and withdrawal symptoms.

Alcohol Dependence Formula:

$$\text{Alcohol Dependence} = \frac{\text{Excessive Consumption} + \text{Physical Dependence}}{\text{Control Loss}}$$

Alcohol dependence is characterized by excessive consumption and physical dependence, forming a ratio relative to the loss of control.

Opioid Equation:

$$\text{Opioid Use Disorder} = \text{Pain Relief} + \text{Euphoria} - \text{Respiratory Depression}$$

Opioid use disorder involves seeking pain relief and euphoria while balancing the risk of respiratory depression.

Dopamine Rollercoaster:

$$\text{Dopamine Rollercoaster} = \text{Reward Seeking} + \text{Hedonic Impact} - \text{Consequences}$$

Addiction takes individuals on a dopamine rollercoaster, driven by reward-seeking behavior and the hedonic impact of substances, often disregarding consequences.

These symbolic equations offer a creative way to represent substance-related and addictive disorders, emphasizing key components and dynamics associated with these conditions.

Chapter 3

Assessment and Diagnosis

3.1 Clinical Interview Techniques

Communication Formula:

$$\text{Communication} = \frac{\text{Active Listening} + \text{Empathy} + \text{Open-ended Questions}}{\text{Distractions}}$$

Effective clinical interviews involve a balance of active listening, empathy, and open-ended questions, minimizing distractions for optimal communication.

Diagnostic Puzzle:

$$\text{Diagnostic Puzzle} = \text{Signs} + \text{Symptoms} + \text{Patient History}$$

The clinical interview is like solving a diagnostic puzzle, piecing together signs, symptoms, and the patient's history for a comprehensive understanding.

RAPPORT Score:

$$\text{RAPPORT} = \text{Rapport Building} + \text{Assessment Precision} + \text{Patient Comfort}$$

The success of a clinical interview can be measured by the RAPPORT score, combining rapport building, assessment precision, and ensuring patient comfort.

Therapeutic Alliance Quotient:

$$\text{Therapeutic Alliance} = \text{Trust} \times \left(\frac{\text{Collaboration}}{\text{Resistance}} \right)$$

Building a therapeutic alliance involves cultivating trust and collaboration while minimizing resistance during the clinical interview.

These symbolic equations offer a creative way to represent clinical interview techniques, emphasizing the essential components and dynamics involved in the assessment and diagnosis process.

3.2 Psychological Testing

Testing Equation:

$$\text{Testing} = \text{Questionnaires} + \text{Observations} + \text{Scores}$$

Psychological testing involves the combination of questionnaires, observations, and scoring mechanisms to assess various aspects of an individual.

IQ Formula:

$$\text{IQ} = \frac{\text{Mental Age}}{\text{Chronological Age}} \times 100$$

IQ, or intelligence quotient, is calculated by dividing mental age by chronological age and multiplying the result by 100.

Personality Chemistry:

$$\text{Personality Chemistry} = \text{Traits} \times \left(\frac{\text{Adaptability}}{\text{Stability}}\right)$$

Personality testing involves exploring traits in a dynamic balance, where adaptability over stability contributes to the individual's unique chemistry.

Anxiety Quotient:

$$\text{Anxiety Quotient} = \frac{\text{Worry Intensity}}{\text{Coping Mechanisms}}$$

Measuring anxiety involves assessing the intensity of worry relative to the effectiveness of an individual's coping mechanisms.

These symbolic equations offer a creative way to represent psychological testing, emphasizing key components and formulas associated with the assessment process.

3.3 Neuroimaging in Psychiatry

Brain Snapshot:

$$\text{Brain Snapshot} = \text{fMRI} + \text{PET} + \text{EEG}$$

Neuroimaging in psychiatry captures a dynamic brain snapshot through functional magnetic resonance imaging (fMRI), positron emission tomography (PET), and electroencephalography (EEG).

Connectivity Matrix:

$$\text{Connectivity Matrix} = \text{Neural Pathways} + \text{Synaptic Strength} + \text{Communication Efficiency}$$

Analyzing neuroimaging data involves constructing a connectivity matrix, integrating neural pathways, synaptic strength, and communication efficiency.

Dopamine Dance:

$$\text{Dopamine Dance} = \text{Dopamine Release} \times \left(\frac{\text{Reuptake}}{\text{Neuronal Excitability}} \right)$$

Neuroimaging unveils the dopamine dance in psychiatric conditions, influenced by dopamine release, reuptake, and neuronal excitability.

Structural Harmony:

$$\text{Structural Harmony} = \text{MRI} + \text{CT} + \text{Neuronal Density}$$

Neuroimaging techniques like magnetic resonance imaging (MRI) and computed tomography (CT) contribute to understanding the structural harmony of the brain, including neuronal density.

These symbolic equations offer a creative way to represent neuroimaging in psychiatry, emphasizing the diverse techniques and the information they reveal about the brain.

3.4 Laboratory Tests

Chemical Equation:

$$\text{Chemical Equation} = \text{Blood Sample} + \text{Biomarkers} + \text{Assay Techniques}$$

Laboratory tests in psychiatry involve a chemical equation, combining blood samples, biomarkers, and assay techniques to unveil crucial information.

Neurotransmitter Formula:

$$\text{Neurotransmitter Levels} = \text{Serotonin} + \text{Dopamine} + \text{Norepinephrine}$$

Assessing neurotransmitter levels reveals insights into psychiatric conditions, where serotonin, dopamine, and norepinephrine play key roles.

Genetic Blueprint:

$$\text{Genetic Blueprint} = \text{DNA Analysis} + \text{Polymorphisms} + \text{Susceptibility Genes}$$

Laboratory tests explore the genetic blueprint through DNA analysis, identifying polymorphisms and susceptibility genes linked to psychiatric disorders.

Hormonal Harmony:

$$\text{Hormonal Harmony} = \text{Hormone Levels} + \text{Feedback Mechanisms} + \text{Endocrine Function}$$

Assessing hormonal harmony involves measuring hormone levels, understanding feedback mechanisms, and evaluating overall endocrine function.

These symbolic equations offer a creative way to represent laboratory tests in psychiatry, emphasizing the diverse methods and information they provide for assessment and diagnosis.

3.5   Differential Diagnosis

Variety Equation:

$$\text{Variety} = \text{Symptom Diversity} + \text{Medical Conditions} + \text{Psychological Factors}$$

Differential diagnosis involves considering a variety of factors, including the diversity of symptoms, medical conditions, and psychological factors.

Commonality Index:

$$\text{Commonality} = \frac{\text{Shared Symptoms}}{\text{Distinct Features}}$$

Evaluating differential diagnoses requires assessing the commonality index, measuring shared symptoms relative to distinct features.

Probability Matrix:

$$\text{Probability Matrix} = \text{Prevalence} \times \text{Specificity} \nabla \cdot \text{Sensitivity}$$

Calculating probabilities involves a matrix of prevalence, specificity, and sensitivity, aiding in the differentiation of potential diagnoses.

Dynamic Algorithm:

$$\text{Dynamic Algorithm} = \text{Iterative Assessment} + \text{Refinement} + \text{Expert Input}$$

Differential diagnosis is a dynamic algorithm, involving iterative assessment, continual refinement, and input from experts for accurate conclusions.

These symbolic equations offer a creative way to represent differential diagnosis, emphasizing the dynamic and multifaceted nature of the process.

3.6 Cultural Considerations in Assessment

Cultural Sensitivity Formula:

$$\text{Cultural Sensitivity} = \frac{\text{Cultural Awareness} + \text{Cultural Competence}}{\text{Stereotype Avoidance}}$$

Cultural considerations in assessment involve enhancing cultural sensitivity by combining cultural awareness and competence while actively avoiding stereotypes.

Diversity Quotient:

$$\text{Diversity Quotient} = \text{Cultural Backgrounds} \times \left(\frac{\text{Language Variability}}{\text{Cultural Relatability}} \right)$$

Assessment should consider a diversity quotient, acknowledging various cultural backgrounds and incorporating language variability relative to cultural relatability.

Inclusivity Index:

$$\text{Inclusivity Index} = \frac{\text{Cultural Representation}}{\text{Exclusionary Practices}}$$

Cultural considerations aim for an inclusivity index, emphasizing cultural representation while minimizing exclusionary practices in assessment.

Cultural Harmony Equation:

$$\text{Cultural Harmony} = \text{Respect} \times \left(\frac{\text{Adaptability}}{\text{Cultural Reciprocity}} \right)$$

Achieving cultural harmony in assessment involves cultivating respect and adaptability, with a focus on reciprocal cultural understanding.

These symbolic equations offer a creative way to represent cultural considerations in assessment, highlighting the importance of cultural sensitivity and inclusivity.

Chapter 4

Treatment Modalities

4.1 Pharmacotherapy

Symptom Equation:

$$\text{Symptom Relief} = \text{Medication Efficacy} \times \left(\frac{\text{Tolerance Development}}{\text{Side Effects}} \right)$$

Pharmacotherapy aims for symptom relief by considering medication efficacy, managing tolerance development, and minimizing side effects.

Neurochemical Harmony:

$$\text{Neuro Harmony} = \text{Receptor Activation} + \text{Neurotransmitter Balance} - \text{Downregulation}$$

Medications seek neurochemical harmony by activating receptors, balancing neurotransmitter levels, and preventing downregulation.

Treatment Compliance Index:

$$\text{Compliance} = \frac{\text{Patient Adherence}}{\text{Medication Complexity} \times \text{Side Effect Burden}}$$

Ensuring treatment compliance involves assessing patient adherence relative to medication complexity and the burden of side effects.

Dose-Response Curve:

$$\text{Response} = \text{Dose} \times \left(\frac{\text{Individual Sensitivity}}{\text{Tolerance Level}} \right)$$

Medication response follows a dose-response curve, influenced by individual sensitivity and tolerance levels.

These symbolic equations offer a creative way to represent pharmacotherapy, emphasizing factors influencing symptom relief and neurochemical balance.

4.2 Psychotherapy Approaches

Therapeutic Equation:

$$\text{Therapeutic Progress} = \text{Therapeutic Alliance} + \text{Insight Gain} + \text{Skill Acquisition}$$

Psychotherapy aims for therapeutic progress, combining the strength of the therapeutic alliance, insight gain, and skill acquisition.

Cognitive Restructuring Formula:

$$\text{Cognitive Restructuring} = \text{Identify Distorted Thoughts} + \text{Challenge Beliefs} + \text{Adopt Rational Thinking}$$

Cognitive restructuring involves identifying distorted thoughts, challenging beliefs, and adopting rational thinking for effective psychotherapeutic outcomes.

Behavioral Activation Index:

$$\text{Behavioral Activation} = \frac{\text{Activity Planning}}{\text{Avoidance Reduction}}$$

Behavioral activation is measured by the index of activity planning relative to the reduction of avoidance behaviors during psychotherapy.

Interpersonal Equation:

$$\text{Interpersonal Effectiveness} = \text{Communication Skills} \times \left(\frac{\text{Empathy}}{\text{Boundary Setting}} \right)$$

Interpersonal effectiveness in psychotherapy involves honing communication skills, emphasizing empathy, and setting appropriate boundaries.

These symbolic equations offer a creative way to represent psychotherapy approaches, emphasizing key elements contributing to therapeutic progress.

4.3 Electroconvulsive Therapy (ECT)

Brain Reset Equation:

$$\text{Brain Reset} = \text{Electrical Pulses} \times \left(\frac{\text{Seizure Induction}}{\text{Neuroplasticity Boost}} \right)$$

ECT involves a "brain reset" achieved by delivering electrical pulses, inducing controlled seizures, and promoting neuroplasticity for therapeutic benefits.

Memory Reconsolidation Formula:

$$\text{Memory Reconsolidation} = \text{Amnesia Induction} \times \left(\frac{\text{Memory Adaptation}}{\text{Trauma Processing}} \right)$$

ECT contributes to memory reconsolidation by inducing amnesia, facilitating memory adaptation, and aiding in trauma processing during therapy.

Neural Network Reconfiguration:

$$\text{Neural Reconfiguration} = \text{Synaptic Connectivity} + \text{Neuronal Excitability} - \text{Depressive Circuit Reset}$$

ECT aims at neural network reconfiguration, enhancing synaptic connectivity, modulating neuronal excitability, and resetting depressive circuits in the brain.

Depression Breakdown:

$$\text{Depression Breakdown} = \text{Chemical Equilibrium} \times \left(\frac{\text{Mood Stabilization}}{\text{Resistant Symptoms}} \right)$$

ECT facilitates a breakdown of depression by restoring chemical equilibrium, stabilizing mood, and addressing resistant symptoms in a therapeutic manner.

These symbolic equations offer a creative way to represent Electroconvulsive Therapy, emphasizing its impact on brain function and its role in treating certain psychiatric conditions.

4.4 Transcranial Magnetic Stimulation (TMS)

Brain Activation Equation:

$$\text{Brain Activation} = \text{TMS Pulses} \times \left(\frac{\text{Neural Excitability}}{\text{Depression Inhibition}} \right)$$

TMS induces brain activation by delivering pulses, enhancing neural excitability, and inhibiting depressive circuits for therapeutic effects.

Cortical Resonance Index:

$$\text{Cortical Resonance} = \text{TMS Frequency} \times \left(\frac{\text{Neuronal Synchronization}}{\text{Maladaptive Connectivity}} \right)$$

TMS modulates cortical resonance through frequency adjustments, promoting neuronal synchronization and disrupting maladaptive connectivity.

Neuroplasticity Boost:

$$\text{Neuroplasticity} = \text{TMS Intensity} \times \left(\frac{\text{Synaptic Plasticity}}{\text{Learning Enhancement}} \right)$$

TMS provides a neuroplasticity boost by adjusting intensity, enhancing synaptic plasticity, and facilitating learning processes.

Mood Oscillation Harmonizer:

$$\text{Mood Oscillation} = \text{TMS Sessions} \times \left(\frac{\text{Stabilization}}{\text{Cyclic Fluctuations}} \right)$$

TMS acts as a mood oscillation harmonizer, stabilizing mood through sessions and mitigating cyclic fluctuations associated with mood disorders.

These symbolic equations offer a creative way to represent Transcranial Magnetic Stimulation, emphasizing its role in modulating brain activity and promoting therapeutic outcomes.

4.5   Neurosurgical Interventions

Lesion Elimination:

$$\text{Lesion Elimination} = \text{Lesion Removal} \times \left(\frac{\text{Functional Restoration}}{\text{Compensatory Mechanisms}} \right)$$

Neurosurgical interventions aim at lesion elimination by removing pathological structures, restoring function, and minimizing reliance on compensatory mechanisms.

Connectivity Restoration:

$$\text{Connectivity Restoration} = \text{Neural Pathway Repair} \times \left(\frac{\text{Synaptic Reconnection}}{\text{Plasticity Enhancement}} \right)$$

Neurosurgery contributes to connectivity restoration by repairing neural pathways, promoting synaptic reconnection, and enhancing neuroplasticity.

Deep Stimulation Equation:

$$\text{Deep Stimulation} = \text{Electrode Insertion} \times \left(\frac{\text{Neural Modulation}}{\text{Symptom Alleviation}} \right)$$

Deep brain stimulation involves electrode insertion, modulating neural activity, and alleviating symptoms through targeted stimulation.

Seizure Circuit Disruption:

$$\text{Seizure Disruption} = \text{Hippocampal Ablation} \times \left(\frac{\text{Seizure Suppression}}{\text{Cognitive Impact Minimization}} \right)$$

For epilepsy treatment, neurosurgery disrupts seizure circuits by ablating the hippocampus, suppressing seizures, and minimizing cognitive impact.

These symbolic equations offer a creative way to represent neurosurgical interventions, emphasizing their role in eliminating lesions, restoring connectivity, and modulating neural function for therapeutic outcomes.

4.6 Complementary and Alternative Therapies

Holistic Harmony Equation:

$$\text{Holistic Harmony} = \text{Mind-Body Connection} \times \left(\frac{\text{Energy Flow}}{\text{Stress Reduction}} \right)$$

Complementary therapies seek holistic harmony by emphasizing the mind-body connection, enhancing energy flow, and reducing stress for overall well-being.

Herbal Efficacy Index:

$$\text{Herbal Efficacy} = \text{Herb Potency} \times \left(\frac{\text{Adaptogenic Properties}}{\text{Symptom Alleviation}} \right)$$

Alternative therapies leverage herbal efficacy, considering potency and adaptogenic properties to alleviate symptoms and promote wellness.

Acupuncture Balance Formula:

$$\text{Acupuncture Balance} = \text{Meridian Alignment} \times \left(\frac{\text{Qi Flow}}{\text{Pain Relief}} \right)$$

Acupuncture aims for balance by aligning meridians, facilitating Qi flow, and providing pain relief through traditional Chinese medicine practices.

Meditative Resonance Quotient:

$$\text{Resonance} = \frac{\text{Mindfulness}}{\text{Relaxation Techniques} \times \text{Breathing Exercises}}$$

Complementary therapies enhance meditative resonance by emphasizing mindfulness, relaxation techniques, and breathing exercises for therapeutic benefits.

These symbolic equations offer a creative way to represent complementary and alternative therapies, emphasizing their holistic nature and diverse approaches to well-being.

Chapter 5

Psychopharmacology

5.1 Introduction to Psychotropic Medications

Synaptic Harmony Equation:

$$\text{Synaptic Harmony} = \text{Neurotransmitter Modulation} \times \left(\frac{\text{Receptor Affinity}}{\text{Neuronal Stabilization}} \right)$$

Psychotropic medications aim for synaptic harmony, modulating neurotransmitters, optimizing receptor affinity, and stabilizing neuronal activity for therapeutic effects.

Mood Equation:

$$\text{Mood} = \text{Serotonin} + \text{Dopamine} + \text{Norepinephrine} + \text{GABA} - \text{Glutamate}$$

Balancing mood involves adjusting the levels of key neurotransmitters - serotonin, dopamine, norepinephrine, GABA, and modulating glutamate.

Dose Titration Index:

$$\text{Dose Titration} = \frac{\text{Clinical Response}}{\text{Side Effect Tolerance}}$$

Optimizing dose titration requires balancing the clinical response with the tolerance of potential side effects to achieve an effective and well-tolerated treatment.

Reuptake Inhibition Quotient:

$$\text{Reuptake Inhibition} = \frac{\text{Neurotransmitter Availability}}{\text{Reuptake Pump Activity}}$$

Some medications exert their effects through reuptake inhibition, altering neurotransmitter availability by modulating reuptake pump activity.

These symbolic equations offer a creative way to represent the introduction to psychotropic medications, emphasizing their role in modulating neurotransmitters and achieving therapeutic outcomes.

5.2   Antidepressants

Serotonin Boost Equation:

$$\text{Serotonin Boost} =$$

Selective Serotonin Reuptake Inhibition (SSRI)+Serotonin-Norepinephrine Reuptake Inhibition (SNRI)

Antidepressants boost serotonin levels through mechanisms like SSRI and SNRI, enhancing synaptic availability for mood regulation.

Neurogenesis Activation:

$$\text{Neurogenesis} = \text{Brain-Derived Neurotrophic Factor (BDNF)} + \text{Hippocampal Plasticity}$$

Certain antidepressants activate neurogenesis by increasing BDNF and promoting hippocampal plasticity, contributing to therapeutic effects.

Monoamine Receptor Modulation:

$$\text{Monoamine Modulation} = \text{Tricyclic Antidepressants (TCA)}+\text{Monoamine Oxidase Inhibitors (MAOI)}$$

TCAs and MAOIs modulate monoamine receptors, altering neurotransmitter activity and influencing mood regulation in antidepressant treatment.

Synaptic Resilience Quotient:

$$\text{Resilience} = \frac{\text{Neuronal Adaptation}}{\text{Synaptic Receptor Sensitivity} \times \text{Cytokine Regulation}}$$

Antidepressants promote synaptic resilience by enhancing neuronal adaptation, modulating receptor sensitivity, and regulating cytokines for mood stabilization.

These symbolic equations offer a creative way to represent antidepressants, emphasizing their diverse mechanisms and impact on neurotransmitter systems for therapeutic benefits.

5.3 Antipsychotics

Dopamine Balance Equation:

$$\text{Dopamine Balance} = \text{D2 Blockade} + \text{Mesocortical Pathway Modulation}$$

Antipsychotics achieve dopamine balance through D2 receptor blockade and modulation of the mesocortical pathway, reducing excessive neurotransmission linked to psychosis.

Serotonin-Dopamine Synergy:

$$\text{Synergy} = \text{5-HT2A Antagonism} + \text{D2 Receptor Control}$$

Optimal antipsychotic effects involve the synergy between serotonin (5-HT2A) antagonism and D2 receptor control, enhancing neurotransmitter balance.

Serenity Quotient:

$$\text{Serenity} = \frac{\text{Dopamine Stabilization}}{\text{Cognitive Impact} \times \text{Extrapyramidal Tolerance}}$$

Antipsychotics aim for a serenity quotient by stabilizing dopamine, managing cognitive impact, and ensuring tolerability of extrapyramidal symptoms.

Neuronal Adaptability Index:

$$\text{Adaptability} = \frac{\text{Neuronal Resilience}}{\text{D2 Sensitivity} \times \text{Anticholinergic Management}}$$

Antipsychotics promote neuronal adaptability by enhancing resilience, adjusting D2 receptor sensitivity, and effectively managing anticholinergic effects.

These symbolic equations offer a creative way to represent antipsychotics, emphasizing their role in achieving neurotransmitter balance and therapeutic outcomes in the treatment of psychotic disorders.

5.4 Mood Stabilizers

Lithium Equilibrium:

$$\text{Lithium Stability} = \text{Neuronal Sodium Transport Inhibition} + \text{GSK-3 Modulation}$$

Mood stabilizers like lithium maintain stability by inhibiting neuronal sodium transport and modulating GSK-3, contributing to therapeutic effects.

Neurotransmitter Harmony:

$$\text{Harmony} = \text{Glutamate Inhibition} + \text{Serotonin Enhancement} + \text{Dopamine Balance}$$

Achieving neurotransmitter harmony involves mood stabilizers inhibiting glutamate, enhancing serotonin, and balancing dopamine for mood regulation.

Calcium Channel Resilience:

$$\text{Resilience} = \frac{\text{Calcium Channel Modulation}}{\text{Neuronal Adaptation} \times \text{Cognitive Stability}}$$

Mood stabilizers enhance resilience by modulating calcium channels, promoting neuronal adaptation, and ensuring cognitive stability for patients.

Intracellular Signaling Quotient:

$$\text{Signaling} = \frac{\text{Inositol Depletion}}{\text{IP3 Kinase Inhibition} \times \text{Cyclic AMP Modulation}}$$

Mood stabilizers influence intracellular signaling by depleting inositol, inhibiting IP3 kinase, and modulating cyclic AMP, contributing to mood stabilization.

These symbolic equations offer a creative way to represent mood stabilizers, emphasizing their mechanisms and impact on neurotransmitters for therapeutic outcomes in mood disorders.

5.5   Anxiolytics and Sedatives

GABAergic Tranquility Equation:

$$\text{GABA Tranquility} = \text{GABA Receptor Activation} + \text{Chloride Influx}$$

Anxiolytics and sedatives induce tranquility by activating GABA receptors, facilitating chloride influx and enhancing inhibitory neurotransmission.

Sedation Harmony Formula:

$$\text{Sedation Harmony} = \frac{\text{Alpha-1 Blockade}}{\text{Histamine H1 Inhibition} \times \text{CNS Depression}}$$

Achieving sedation harmony involves blocking alpha-1 receptors, inhibiting histamine H1 receptors, and inducing central nervous system (CNS) depression.

Benzodiazepine Potency Index:

$$\text{Potency} = \text{Benzodiazepine Binding} \times \left(\frac{\text{Sedative Strength}}{\text{Tolerance Risk}} \right)$$

Anxiolytics with benzodiazepine affinity exhibit potency by binding to receptors, delivering sedative strength while managing the risk of tolerance development.

Serotonin-GABA Synergy Quotient:

$$\text{Synergy} = \text{Serotonin (5-HT1A) Activation} + \text{GABAergic Modulation}$$

Some anxiolytics enhance tranquility through serotonin (5-HT1A) activation, synergizing with GABAergic modulation for anxiolysis and sedation.

These symbolic equations offer a creative way to represent anxiolytics and sedatives, emphasizing their mechanisms and impact on neurotransmitters for therapeutic outcomes in anxiety and sedation.

5.6 Side Effects and Monitoring

Side Effect Risk Equation:

$$\text{Side Effect Risk} = \text{Metabolism Rate} \times \left(\frac{\text{Blood-Brain Barrier Permeability}}{\text{Liver Enzyme Induction}} \right)$$

The risk of side effects is influenced by the metabolism rate, blood-brain barrier permeability, and the potential for liver enzyme induction.

Tolerability Quotient:

$$\text{Tolerability} = \frac{\text{Clinical Efficacy}}{\text{Adverse Effects Severity} \times \text{Patient Compliance}}$$

Optimizing tolerability involves balancing clinical efficacy with the severity of adverse effects and patient compliance.

Genetic Susceptibility Index:

$$\text{Susceptibility} = \text{Genetic Variants} \times \left(\frac{\text{Drug Metabolism Rate}}{\text{Receptor Sensitivity}} \right)$$

Monitoring for genetic susceptibility considers variants influencing drug metabolism rate and receptor sensitivity.

Serotonin Syndrome Risk:

$$\text{Serotonin Syndrome Risk} = \text{Serotonin Enhancers} \times \left(\frac{\text{CYP450 Inhibition}}{\text{Temperature Dysregulation}} \right)$$

Monitoring serotonin syndrome risk involves assessing serotonin enhancers, CYP450 inhibition potential, and susceptibility to temperature dysregulation.

These symbolic equations offer a creative way to represent side effects and monitoring, emphasizing factors influencing side effect risk, tolerability, genetic susceptibility, and specific risks such as serotonin syndrome.

Chapter 6

Child and Adolescent Psychiatry

6.1 Developmental Considerations

Neuroplasticity Growth Formula:

$$\text{Neuroplasticity Growth} = \text{Environmental Stimulation} \times \left(\frac{\text{Learning Opportunities}}{\text{Cognitive Flexibility}} \right)$$

Child and adolescent development thrive on neuroplasticity growth, influenced by environmental stimulation, learning opportunities, and cognitive flexibility.

Emotional Resilience Index:

$$\text{Resilience} = \frac{\text{Emotional Support}}{\text{Adversity Coping Skills} \times \text{Social Connection}}$$

Promoting emotional resilience involves providing support, enhancing coping skills for adversity, and fostering social connections during development.

Psychosocial Milestones Equation:

$$\text{Milestones} = \text{Genetic Factors} \times \left(\frac{\text{Environmental Influences}}{\text{Cultural Context}} \right)$$

Understanding psychosocial milestones considers genetic factors, environmental influences, and the cultural context shaping the developmental trajectory.

Neurotransmitter Maturation Quotient:

$$\text{Maturation} = \text{Dopamine Receptor Development} \times \left(\frac{\text{Serotonin Synthesis}}{\text{GABAergic Modulation}} \right)$$

Assessing neurotransmitter maturation involves evaluating dopamine receptor development, serotonin synthesis, and GABAergic modulation during development.

These symbolic equations offer a creative way to represent developmental considerations in child and adolescent psychiatry, emphasizing the complex interplay of factors influencing growth, resilience, psychosocial milestones, and neurotransmitter maturation.

6.2   Common Childhood Disorders

Attention Balance Equation:

$$\text{Attention Balance} = \text{Dopamine Dysfunction} \times \left(\frac{\text{Executive Function Impairment}}{\text{Sensory Overload}} \right)$$

Common childhood disorders often involve attention balance affected by dopamine dysfunction, executive function impairment, and sensory overload.

Mood Swing Oscillation:

$$\text{Mood Oscillation} = \text{Genetic Predisposition} \times \left(\frac{\text{Stress Exposure}}{\text{Emotional Regulation Capacity}} \right)$$

Understanding mood swings in childhood disorders considers genetic predisposition, stress exposure, and the capacity for emotional regulation.

Anxiety Sensitivity Index:

$$\text{Sensitivity} = \frac{\text{Anxiety Triggers}}{\text{Coping Mechanisms} \times \text{Resilience Factors}}$$

Common childhood anxiety is influenced by an anxiety sensitivity index, considering triggers, coping mechanisms, and resilience factors.

Neurodevelopmental Harmony:

$$\text{Harmony} = \text{Neurotransmitter Balance} \times \left(\frac{\text{Brain Maturation}}{\text{Genetic-Environmental Interplay}} \right)$$

Neurodevelopmental disorders involve seeking harmony, balancing neurotransmitters, supporting brain maturation, and understanding genetic-environmental interplay.

These symbolic equations offer a creative way to represent common childhood disorders in child and adolescent psychiatry, emphasizing factors impacting attention, mood, anxiety, and neurodevelopmental harmony.

6.3 School-Related Issues

Academic Performance Equation:

$$\text{Academic Performance} = \text{Cognitive Function} \times \left(\frac{\text{Emotional Well-being}}{\text{Attention Regulation}} \right)$$

School-related issues often revolve around academic performance influenced by cognitive function, emotional well-being, and attention regulation.

Social Integration Index:

$$\text{Integration} = \frac{\text{Social Skills}}{\text{Peer Relationship Quality} \times \text{Bullying Exposure}}$$

Understanding social issues involves assessing the social integration index, considering social skills, peer relationship quality, and exposure to bullying.

School Stress Resilience Quotient:

$$\text{Resilience} = \frac{\text{Stress Coping Abilities}}{\text{Supportive School Environment} \times \text{Adaptability}}$$

Managing school-related stress requires evaluating the school stress resilience quotient, including coping abilities, a supportive environment, and adaptability.

Educational Motivation Harmony:

$$\text{Harmony} = \text{Intrinsic Motivation} \times \left(\frac{\text{Parental Involvement}}{\text{Learning Disabilities}} \right)$$

Addressing school-related issues involves achieving educational motivation harmony, balancing intrinsic motivation, parental involvement, and addressing learning disabilities.

These symbolic equations offer a creative way to represent school-related issues in child and adolescent psychiatry, emphasizing factors impacting academic performance, social integration, stress resilience, and educational motivation.

6.4 Family Dynamics

Communication Synchrony Index:

$$\text{Communication Synchrony} = \text{Effective Communication} \times \left(\frac{\text{Conflict Resolution Skills}}{\text{Emotional Support}} \right)$$

Family dynamics can be assessed using the communication synchrony index, incorporating effective communication, conflict resolution skills, and emotional support.

Emotional Climate Equation:

$$\text{Emotional Climate} = \frac{\text{Expressed Emotions}}{\text{Empathy Level} \times \text{Parental Involvement}}$$

Understanding family dynamics involves evaluating the emotional climate, considering expressed emotions, empathy levels, and parental involvement.

Attachment Security Quotient:

$$\text{Attachment Security} = \text{Secure Attachment Bonds} \times \left(\frac{\text{Autonomy Encouragement}}{\text{Parental Consistency}} \right)$$

Assessing family relationships includes the attachment security quotient, combining secure attachment bonds, autonomy encouragement, and parental consistency.

Resilient Family Dynamics:

$$\text{Resilience} = \frac{\text{Adaptive Coping Strategies}}{\text{Family Cohesion} \times \text{Open Communication}}$$

Promoting resilient family dynamics involves fostering adaptive coping strategies, family cohesion, and open communication.

These symbolic equations offer a creative way to represent family dynamics in child and adolescent psychiatry, emphasizing factors impacting communication, emotional climate, attachment security, and resilience within the family unit.

6.5   Intervention Strategies

Therapeutic Alliance Equation:

$$\text{Therapeutic Alliance} = \text{Trust Building} \times \left(\frac{\text{Empathetic Understanding}}{\text{Collaborative Goal Setting}} \right)$$

Effective intervention strategies rely on building a therapeutic alliance, incorporating trust building, empathetic understanding, and collaborative goal setting.

Behavioral Modification Formula:

$$\text{Behavior Modification} = \frac{\text{Positive Reinforcement}}{\text{Consistent Consequences} \times \text{Individualized Plans}}$$

Behavioral interventions involve utilizing the behavioral modification formula, incorporating positive reinforcement, consistent consequences, and individualized plans.

Cognitive Restructuring Quotient:

$$\text{Restructuring} = \text{Cognitive Reframing} \times \left(\frac{\text{Thought-Challenging Techniques}}{\text{Mindfulness Practices}} \right)$$

Cognitive interventions consider the cognitive restructuring quotient, emphasizing cognitive reframing, thought-challenging techniques, and mindfulness practices.

Expressive Arts Therapy Index:

$$\text{Expressive Arts Therapy} = \frac{\text{Creative Expression}}{\text{Emotional Release} \times \text{Therapeutic Processing}}$$

Incorporating expressive arts therapy involves assessing the expressive arts therapy index, considering creative expression, emotional release, and therapeutic processing.

These symbolic equations offer a creative way to represent intervention strategies in child and adolescent psychiatry, emphasizing the importance of therapeutic alliance, behavioral modification, cognitive restructuring, and expressive arts therapy.

6.6 Preventive Measures

Resilience Building Equation:

$$\text{Resilience Building} = \text{Positive Role Modeling} \times \left(\frac{\text{Coping Skills Education}}{\text{Social Support Networks}} \right)$$

Preventive measures involve resilience building, combining positive role modeling, coping skills education, and social support networks.

Preventive Lifestyle Index:

$$\text{Lifestyle} = \frac{\text{Healthy Habits}}{\text{Stress Management} \times \text{Sleep Hygiene}}$$

Incorporating preventive lifestyle measures includes the preventive lifestyle index, focusing on healthy habits, stress management, and sleep hygiene.

Community Involvement Quotient:

$$\text{Involvement} = \text{Community Engagement} \times \left(\frac{\text{Mentorship Programs}}{\text{Access to Resources}} \right)$$

Community involvement plays a role in preventive measures, with the community involvement quotient considering engagement, mentorship programs, and access to resources.

Educational Resilience Formula:

$$\text{Educational Resilience} = \frac{\text{Early Intervention}}{\text{Anti-Bullying Initiatives} \times \text{School Support Systems}}$$

Promoting educational resilience involves the educational resilience formula, incorporating early intervention, anti-bullying initiatives, and school support systems.

These symbolic equations offer a creative way to represent preventive measures in child and adolescent psychiatry, emphasizing the importance of resilience building, lifestyle factors, community involvement, and educational resilience.

Chapter 7

Geriatric Psychiatry

7.1 Aging and Mental Health

Cognitive Reserve Equation:

$$\text{Cognitive Reserve} = \text{Lifelong Learning} \times \left(\frac{\text{Brain Reserve Capacity}}{\text{Social Engagement}} \right)$$

Aging and mental health are influenced by the cognitive reserve, combining lifelong learning, brain reserve capacity, and social engagement.

Neurotransmitter Balance Index:

$$\text{Neurotransmitter Balance} = \frac{\text{Dopamine Regulation}}{\text{Serotonin Homeostasis} \times \text{GABAergic Modulation}}$$

Understanding mental health in the elderly involves assessing the neurotransmitter balance index, considering dopamine regulation, serotonin homeostasis, and GABAergic modulation.

Emotional Wellness Quotient:

$$\text{Emotional Wellness} = \text{Emotional Expression} \times \left(\frac{\text{Resilience Factors}}{\text{Stress Management}} \right)$$

Maintaining mental health in aging includes the emotional wellness quotient, emphasizing emotional expression, resilience factors, and stress management.

Social Connection Harmony:

$$\text{Social Connection} = \frac{\text{Social Networks}}{\text{Loneliness Reduction} \times \text{Community Involvement}}$$

Promoting mental health in the elderly involves achieving social connection harmony, balancing social networks, loneliness reduction, and community involvement.

These symbolic equations offer a creative way to represent aging and mental health in geriatric psychiatry, emphasizing cognitive reserve, neurotransmitter balance, emotional wellness, and social connection.

7.2   Common Geriatric Syndromes

Mobility Resilience Equation:

$$\text{Mobility Resilience} = \text{Muscle Strength} \times \left(\frac{\text{Balance Stability}}{\text{Joint Flexibility}} \right)$$

Common geriatric syndromes often involve mobility resilience, influenced by muscle strength, balance stability, and joint flexibility.

Cognition Agility Index:

$$\text{Cognition Agility} = \frac{\text{Memory Retention}}{\text{Processing Speed} \times \text{Executive Function}}$$

Understanding geriatric cognitive syndromes includes the cognition agility index, assessing memory retention, processing speed, and executive function.

Mood Harmony Quotient:

$$\text{Mood Harmony} = \text{Emotional Regulation} \times \left(\frac{\text{Stress Coping Abilities}}{\text{Social Support Networks}} \right)$$

Geriatric syndromes impacting mood are evaluated using the mood harmony quotient, incorporating emotional regulation, stress coping abilities, and social support networks.

Sensory Integration Index:

$$\text{Sensory Integration} = \frac{\text{Vision Acuity}}{\text{Hearing Precision} \times \text{Tactile Sensitivity}}$$

Assessing geriatric syndromes involves the sensory integration index, considering vision acuity, hearing precision, and tactile sensitivity.

These symbolic equations offer a creative way to represent common geriatric syndromes in geriatric psychiatry, emphasizing factors impacting mobility, cognition, mood, and sensory integration.

7.3 Cognitive Disorders in the Elderly

Memory Recall Equation:

$$\text{Memory Recall} = \text{Neurotransmitter Function} \times \left(\frac{\text{Synaptic Plasticity}}{\text{Hippocampal Volume}} \right)$$

Cognitive disorders in the elderly often involve memory recall influenced by neurotransmitter function, synaptic plasticity, and hippocampal volume.

Attention Span Index:

$$\text{Attention Span} = \frac{\text{Dopaminergic Modulation}}{\text{Frontal Lobe Activation} \times \text{Cerebral Blood Flow}}$$

Understanding cognitive disorders includes the attention span index, assessing dopaminergic modulation, frontal lobe activation, and cerebral blood flow.

Executive Function Harmony:

$$\text{Executive Function} = \text{Prefrontal Cortex Health} \times \left(\frac{\text{Working Memory Capacity}}{\text{Inhibitory Control}} \right)$$

Cognitive disorders impact executive function, emphasizing prefrontal cortex health, working memory capacity, and inhibitory control.

Neuroplasticity Support Quotient:

$$\text{Neuroplasticity Support} = \frac{\text{Environmental Stimulation}}{\text{Cognitive Training} \times \text{Social Engagement}}$$

Promoting cognitive health involves the neuroplasticity support quotient, balancing environmental stimulation, cognitive training, and social engagement.

These symbolic equations offer a creative way to represent cognitive disorders in the elderly in geriatric psychiatry, emphasizing factors impacting memory recall, attention span, executive function, and neuroplasticity support.

7.4 Long-Term Care Considerations

Functional Independence Equation:

$$\text{Functional Independence} = \text{Physical Health} \times \left(\frac{\text{Cognitive Abilities}}{\text{Emotional Well-being}} \right)$$

Long-term care considerations involve functional independence, combining physical health, cognitive abilities, and emotional well-being.

Medication Adherence Index:

$$\text{Medication Adherence} = \frac{\text{Health Literacy}}{\text{Routine Integration} \times \text{Social Support}}$$

Managing long-term care includes the medication adherence index, assessing health literacy, routine integration, and social support.

Quality of Life Harmony:

$$\text{Quality of Life} = \text{Life Satisfaction} \times \left(\frac{\text{Social Connectedness}}{\text{Spiritual Well-being}}\right)$$

Providing quality long-term care involves the quality of life harmony, balancing life satisfaction, social connectedness, and spiritual well-being.

Adaptive Living Support Quotient:

$$\text{Adaptive Living Support} = \frac{\text{Caregiver Assistance}}{\text{Home Accessibility} \times \text{Community Resources}}$$

Promoting long-term care includes the adaptive living support quotient, considering caregiver assistance, home accessibility, and community resources.

These symbolic equations offer a creative way to represent long-term care considerations in geriatric psychiatry, emphasizing factors impacting functional independence, medication adherence, quality of life, and adaptive living support.

7.5   End-of-Life Care

Comfort Symmetry Equation:

$$\text{Comfort Symmetry} = \text{Pain Management} \times \left(\frac{\text{Emotional Support}}{\text{Spiritual Well-being}}\right)$$

End-of-life care involves comfort symmetry, combining pain management, emotional support, and spiritual well-being.

Life Reflection Index:

$$\text{Life Reflection} = \frac{\text{Life Review}}{\text{Legacy Building} \times \text{Closure Facilitation}}$$

Facilitating end-of-life discussions includes the life reflection index, assessing life review, legacy building, and closure facilitation.

Dignity Preservation Quotient:

$$\text{Dignity Preservation} = \text{Autonomy Respect} \times \left(\frac{\text{Respectful Communication}}{\text{Cultural Sensitivity}}\right)$$

Providing end-of-life dignity involves the dignity preservation quotient, emphasizing autonomy respect, respectful communication, and cultural sensitivity.

Support Network Harmony:

$$\text{Support Network} = \frac{\text{Family Involvement}}{\text{Care Coordination} \times \text{Bereavement Support}}$$

End-of-life care considers support network harmony, balancing family involvement, care coordination, and bereavement support.

These symbolic equations offer a creative way to represent end-of-life care in geriatric psychiatry, emphasizing factors impacting comfort, life reflection, dignity preservation, and support networks.

7.6 Legal and Ethical Issues

Autonomy Protection Equation:

$$\text{Autonomy Protection} = \text{Informed Consent} \times \left(\frac{\text{Advance Directives}}{\text{Capacity Assessment}} \right)$$

Addressing legal and ethical issues involves autonomy protection, combining informed consent, advance directives, and capacity assessment.

Confidentiality Safeguard Index:

$$\text{Confidentiality Safeguard} = \frac{\text{Privacy Protection}}{\text{Information Sharing Limitations} \times \text{Legal Competence}}$$

Managing legal and ethical considerations includes the confidentiality safeguard index, assessing privacy protection, information sharing limitations, and legal competence.

Beneficence-Focused Harmony:

$$\text{Beneficence-Focused} = \text{Patient Well-being} \times \left(\frac{\text{Risk-Benefit Evaluation}}{\text{Cultural Competency}} \right)$$

Providing ethical care involves the beneficence-focused harmony, balancing patient well-being, risk-benefit evaluation, and cultural competency.

Justice Equity Quotient:

$$\text{Justice Equity} = \frac{\text{Fair Treatment}}{\text{Resource Allocation} \times \text{Legal Advocacy}}$$

Geriatric psychiatry ethics considers the justice equity quotient, promoting fair treatment, responsible resource allocation, and legal advocacy.

These symbolic equations offer a creative way to represent legal and ethical issues in geriatric psychiatry, emphasizing factors impacting autonomy protection, confidentiality safeguard, beneficence-focused care, and justice equity.

Chapter 8

Forensic Psychiatry

8.1 Legal Standards in Psychiatry

Criminal Responsibility Index:

$$\text{Criminal Responsibility} = \text{Mental State at Offense} \times \left(\frac{\text{Insanity Assessment}}{\text{Volitional Impairment}} \right)$$

Evaluating criminal responsibility involves the criminal responsibility index, considering the mental state at the offense, insanity assessment, and volitional impairment.

Competency to Stand Trial Equation:

$$\text{Competency to Stand Trial} = \frac{\text{Understanding Legal Proceedings}}{\text{Assistance in Defense} \times \text{Courtroom Behavior}}$$

Assessing competency to stand trial includes the competency to stand trial equation, evaluating understanding of legal proceedings, assistance in defense, and courtroom behavior.

Risk Assessment Quotient:

$$\text{Risk Assessment} = \text{Potential for Harm} \times \left(\frac{\text{Protective Factors}}{\text{Previous Criminal History}} \right)$$

Legal standards in forensic psychiatry involve risk assessment, combining potential for harm, protective factors, and previous criminal history.

Sentencing Recommendation Harmony:

$$\text{Sentencing Recommendation} = \frac{\text{Rehabilitation Potential}}{\text{Public Safety Considerations} \times \text{Reintegration Plan}}$$

Providing legal standards considers the sentencing recommendation harmony, balancing rehabilitation potential, public safety considerations, and reintegration plans.

These symbolic equations offer a creative way to represent legal standards in forensic psychiatry, emphasizing factors impacting criminal responsibility, competency to stand trial, risk assessment, and sentencing recommendations.

8.2   Criminal Responsibility

Legal Sanity Quotient:

$$\text{Legal Sanity} = \text{Mental State Evaluation} \times \left(\frac{\text{Insanity Test Outcome}}{\text{Intent Recognition}} \right)$$

Determining criminal responsibility involves the legal sanity quotient, considering mental state evaluation, insanity test outcome, and intent recognition.

Temporal Culpability Index:

$$\text{Temporal Culpability} = \frac{\text{Time of Offense Circumstances}}{\text{Impaired Decision-Making} \times \text{Awareness of Consequences}}$$

Assessing criminal responsibility includes the temporal culpability index, evaluating time of offense circumstances, impaired decision-making, and awareness of consequences.

Cognitive Volition Harmony:

$$\text{Cognitive Volition} = \text{Cognitive Functionality} \times \left(\frac{\text{Volitional Capacity}}{\text{Choice Rationality}} \right)$$

Understanding criminal responsibility involves the cognitive volition harmony, combining cognitive functionality, volitional capacity, and choice rationality.

Intent-Mitigation Factor:

$$\text{Intent-Mitigation} = \frac{\text{Mental Impairment Severity}}{\text{Coercive Factors} \times \text{Substance Influence}}$$

Evaluating criminal responsibility considers the intent-mitigation factor, assessing mental impairment severity, coercive factors, and substance influence.

These symbolic equations offer a creative way to represent criminal responsibility in forensic psychiatry, emphasizing factors impacting legal sanity, temporal culpability, cognitive volition, and intent mitigation.

8.3 Competency and Guardianship

Legal Capacity Quotient:

$$\text{Legal Capacity} = \text{Decisional Competence} \times \left(\frac{\text{Informed Consent Ability}}{\text{Competency Restoration Potential}} \right)$$

Assessing competency involves the legal capacity quotient, combining decisional competence, informed consent ability, and competency restoration potential.

Guardianship Necessity Index:

$$\text{Guardianship Necessity} = \frac{\text{Risk of Harm to Self or Others}}{\text{Functional Impairment} \times \text{Decisional Incapacity}}$$

Determining the need for guardianship includes the guardianship necessity index, evaluating the risk of harm to self or others, functional impairment, and decisional incapacity.

Autonomy-Support Harmony:

$$\text{Autonomy-Support} = \text{Least Restrictive Alternative} \times \left(\frac{\text{Wishes and Preferences Acknowledgment}}{\text{Court Approval Considerations}} \right)$$

Balancing competency and guardianship involves the autonomy-support harmony, emphasizing the least restrictive alternative, acknowledgment of wishes and preferences, and court approval considerations.

Decisional Independence Quotient:

$$\text{Decisional Independence} = \frac{\text{Self-Determination Capacity}}{\text{Risk Management Strategies} \times \text{Surrogate Decision-Making}}$$

Providing support for decision-making considers the decisional independence quotient, assessing self-determination capacity, risk management strategies, and surrogate decision-making.

These symbolic equations offer a creative way to represent competency and guardianship in forensic psychiatry, emphasizing factors impacting legal capacity, guardianship necessity, autonomy-support, and decisional independence.

8.4 Risk Assessment

Danger Potential Equation:

$$\text{Danger Potential} = \text{Risk Factors Severity} \times \left(\frac{\text{Protective Elements}}{\text{Previous Aggression}} \right)$$

Assessing risk involves the danger potential equation, considering the severity of risk factors, protective elements, and previous aggression.

Recidivism Probability Index:

$$\text{Recidivism Probability} = \frac{\text{Criminogenic Factors}}{\text{Rehabilitation Efforts} \times \text{Social Integration}}$$

Evaluating the risk of recidivism includes the recidivism probability index, assessing criminogenic factors, rehabilitation efforts, and social integration.

Threat Level Harmony:

$$\text{Threat Level} = \text{Violence History} \times \left(\frac{\text{Mental Health Stability}}{\text{Stressor Load}} \right)$$

Assessing risk levels involves the threat level harmony, balancing violence history, mental health stability, and stressor load.

Community Safety Quotient:

$$\text{Community Safety} = \frac{\text{Supervision Effectiveness}}{\text{Treatment Compliance} \times \text{Support Network Strength}}$$

Promoting community safety considers the community safety quotient, assessing the effectiveness of supervision, treatment compliance, and support network strength.

These symbolic equations offer a creative way to represent risk assessment in forensic psychiatry, emphasizing factors impacting danger potential, recidivism probability, threat level, and community safety.

8.5   Expert Witness Testimony

Forensic Proficiency Index:

$$\text{Forensic Proficiency} = \text{Clinical Expertise} \times \left(\frac{\text{Legal Knowledge}}{\text{Communication Skills}} \right)$$

Providing expert witness testimony involves the forensic proficiency index, combining clinical expertise, legal knowledge, and communication skills.

Testimonial Impact Quotient:

$$\text{Testimonial Impact} = \frac{\text{Persuasive Testimony}}{\text{Cross-Examination Resilience} \times \text{Jury Perception}}$$

Assessing the impact of testimony includes the testimonial impact quotient, evaluating persuasive testimony, cross-examination resilience, and jury perception.

Credibility Harmony Equation:

$$\text{Credibility Harmony} = \text{Professional Integrity} \times \left(\frac{\text{Empathy Towards the Court}}{\text{Objectivity Maintenance}} \right)$$

Expert witness credibility involves the credibility harmony equation, emphasizing professional integrity, empathy towards the court, and objectivity maintenance.

Data Interpretation Synchrony:

$$\text{Data Interpretation} = \frac{\text{Forensic Analysis Skills}}{\text{Complexity Simplification} \times \text{Clarity in Reporting}}$$

Conveying complex information requires data interpretation synchrony, considering forensic analysis skills, complexity simplification, and clarity in reporting.

These symbolic equations offer a creative way to represent expert witness testimony in forensic psychiatry, emphasizing factors impacting forensic proficiency, testimonial impact, credibility harmony, and data interpretation synchrony.

8.6 Correctional Psychiatry

Incarceration Wellness Index:

$$\text{Incarceration Wellness} = \text{Mental Health Support} \times \left(\frac{\text{Rehabilitation Engagement}}{\text{Crisis Intervention Strategies}} \right)$$

Addressing mental health in correctional settings involves the incarceration wellness index, combining mental health support, rehabilitation engagement, and crisis intervention strategies.

Security-Mental Health Equilibrium:

$$\text{Security-Mental Health} = \frac{\text{Institutional Safety}}{\text{Therapeutic Interventions} \times \text{Inmate Well-being}}$$

Maintaining a balance in correctional psychiatry includes the security-mental health equilibrium, assessing institutional safety, therapeutic interventions, and inmate well-being.

Recidivism Prevention Quotient:

$$\text{Recidivism Prevention} = \text{Reintegration Programs} \times \left(\frac{\text{Community Support}}{\text{Risk Factor Mitigation}} \right)$$

Working towards reducing recidivism involves the recidivism prevention quotient, combining reintegration programs, community support, and risk factor mitigation.

Rehabilitative Justice Harmony:

$$\text{Rehabilitative Justice} = \frac{\text{Correctional Treatment}}{\text{Inmate Accountability} \times \text{Legal Advocacy}}$$

Correctional psychiatry aims for rehabilitative justice harmony, balancing correctional treatment, inmate accountability, and legal advocacy.

These symbolic equations offer a creative way to represent correctional psychiatry in forensic psychiatry, emphasizing factors impacting incarceration wellness, security-mental health equilibrium, recidivism prevention, and rehabilitative justice.

Chapter 9

Community Psychiatry

9.1 Community Mental Health Services

Accessibility Quotient:

$$\text{Accessibility} = \text{Geographic Proximity} \times \left(\frac{\text{Cultural Competency}}{\text{Financial Affordability}} \right)$$

Ensuring accessibility to mental health services involves the accessibility quotient, combining geographic proximity, cultural competency, and financial affordability.

Preventive Outreach Equation:

$$\text{Preventive Outreach} = \frac{\text{Community Education}}{\text{Early Intervention Strategies} \times \text{Stigma Reduction}}$$

Promoting preventive mental health care includes the preventive outreach equation, assessing community education, early intervention strategies, and stigma reduction.

Holistic Wellness Harmony:

$$\text{Holistic Wellness} = \text{Integrated Care Models} \times \left(\frac{\text{Social Support Networks}}{\text{Individual Empowerment}} \right)$$

Community mental health services focus on holistic wellness harmony, combining integrated care models, social support networks, and individual empowerment.

Equitable Resource Allocation:

$$\text{Resource Allocation} = \frac{\text{Service Demand}}{\text{Population Needs Assessment} \times \text{Crisis Management Preparedness}}$$

Providing mental health resources involves equitable resource allocation, considering service demand, population needs assessment, and crisis management preparedness.

These symbolic equations offer a creative way to represent community mental health services in community psychiatry, emphasizing factors impacting accessibility, preventive outreach, holistic wellness, and resource allocation.

9.2   Homelessness and Mental Illness

Vulnerability Index:

$$\text{Vulnerability} = \text{Housing Instability} \times \left(\frac{\text{Psychosocial Stressors}}{\text{Access to Mental Health Resources}} \right)$$

Understanding the vulnerability of individuals involves the vulnerability index, combining housing instability, psychosocial stressors, and access to mental health resources.

Resilience Factor Equation:

$$\text{Resilience Factor} = \frac{\text{Community Support}}{\text{Individual Coping Strategies} \times \text{Employment Stability}}$$

Addressing homelessness and mental illness includes the resilience factor equation, evaluating community support, individual coping strategies, and employment stability.

Trauma-Informed Care Harmony:

$$\text{Trauma-Informed Care} = \text{Trauma History Recognition} \times \left(\frac{\text{Safe Shelter Environments}}{\text{Cultural Sensitivity}} \right)$$

Providing care for those experiencing homelessness and mental illness involves trauma-informed care harmony, combining trauma history recognition, safe shelter environments, and cultural sensitivity.

Housing-Health Symbiosis:

$$\text{Housing-Health} = \frac{\text{Stable Housing}}{\text{Mental Health Stability} \times \text{Substance Use Support}}$$

Promoting stability requires the housing-health symbiosis, assessing stable housing, mental health stability, and substance use support.

These symbolic equations offer a creative way to represent the connection between homelessness and mental illness in community psychiatry, emphasizing factors impacting vulnerability, resilience, trauma-informed care, and housing-health symbiosis.

9.3 Crisis Intervention

Rapid Stabilization Index:

$$\text{Rapid Stabilization} = \text{Assessment Precision} \times \left(\frac{\text{Immediate Support Availability}}{\text{Collaborative Crisis Planning}}\right)$$

Responding to crises involves the rapid stabilization index, combining assessment precision, immediate support availability, and collaborative crisis planning.

De-escalation Efficiency Quotient:

$$\text{De-escalation Efficiency} = \frac{\text{Communication Effectiveness}}{\text{Emotional Regulation Skills} \times \text{Risk Assessment Accuracy}}$$

Efficiently de-escalating crises includes the de-escalation efficiency quotient, evaluating communication effectiveness, emotional regulation skills, and risk assessment accuracy.

Empathetic Intervention Harmony:

$$\text{Empathetic Intervention} = \text{Cultural Competence} \times \left(\frac{\text{Trauma-Informed Practices}}{\text{Client-Centered Approach}}\right)$$

Providing empathetic crisis intervention involves the empathetic intervention harmony, combining cultural competence, trauma-informed practices, and a client-centered approach.

Collaborative Care Synchrony:

$$\text{Collaborative Care} = \frac{\text{Multidisciplinary Team Collaboration}}{\text{Community Resources Accessibility} \times \text{Follow-up Support}}$$

Implementing crisis intervention strategies involves collaborative care synchrony, assessing multidisciplinary team collaboration, community resources accessibility, and follow-up support.

These symbolic equations offer a creative way to represent crisis intervention in community psychiatry, emphasizing factors impacting rapid stabilization, de-escalation efficiency, empathetic intervention, and collaborative care.

9.4 Rehabilitation Programs

Reintegration Success Index:

$$\text{Reintegration Success} = \text{Skill Development} \times \left(\frac{\text{Social Inclusion}}{\text{Employment Stability}}\right)$$

Measuring the success of rehabilitation programs involves the reintegration success index, combining skill development, social inclusion, and employment stability.

Therapeutic Engagement Equation:

$$\text{Therapeutic Engagement} = \frac{\text{Client Motivation}}{\text{Program Adaptability} \times \text{Counseling Effectiveness}}$$

Facilitating therapeutic engagement includes the therapeutic engagement equation, evaluating client motivation, program adaptability, and counseling effectiveness.

Skill Mastery Harmony:

$$\text{Skill Mastery} = \text{Training Consistency} \times \left(\frac{\text{Peer Support}}{\text{Self-Efficacy}}\right)$$

Enhancing skills in rehabilitation programs involves skill mastery harmony, combining training consistency, peer support, and self-efficacy.

Holistic Recovery Quotient:

$$\text{Holistic Recovery} = \frac{\text{Physical Wellness}}{\text{Emotional Resilience} \times \text{Community Integration}}$$

Fostering holistic recovery requires the holistic recovery quotient, assessing physical wellness, emotional resilience, and community integration.

These symbolic equations offer a creative way to represent rehabilitation programs in community psychiatry, emphasizing factors impacting reintegration success, therapeutic engagement, skill mastery, and holistic recovery.

9.5   Preventive Psychiatry

Mental Wellness Prophylaxis:

$$\text{Mental Wellness} = \text{Psychoeducation} \times \left(\frac{\text{Resilience Building}}{\text{Early Intervention Strategies}}\right)$$

Promoting mental wellness involves the mental wellness prophylaxis, combining psychoeducation, resilience building, and early intervention strategies.

Stress Resilience Equation:

$$\text{Stress Resilience} = \frac{\text{Coping Mechanisms}}{\text{Social Support} \times \text{Mindfulness Practices}}$$

Enhancing stress resilience includes the stress resilience equation, evaluating coping mechanisms, social support, and mindfulness practices.

Community Awareness Harmony:

$$\text{Community Awareness} = \text{Public Mental Health Campaigns} \times \left(\frac{\text{Stigma Reduction}}{\text{Accessible Resources}}\right)$$

Fostering community awareness in preventive psychiatry involves community awareness harmony, combining public mental health campaigns, stigma reduction, and accessible resources.

Well-Being Immunity Quotient:

$$\text{Well-Being Immunity} = \frac{\text{Positive Lifestyle Choices}}{\text{Psychosocial Stressors} \times \text{Therapeutic Outlets}}$$

Building well-being immunity requires the well-being immunity quotient, assessing positive lifestyle choices, psychosocial stressors, and therapeutic outlets.

These symbolic equations offer a creative way to represent preventive psychiatry in community psychiatry, emphasizing factors impacting mental wellness, stress resilience, community awareness, and well-being immunity.

9.6 Public Policy and Advocacy

Policy Impact Index:

$$\text{Policy Impact} = \text{Legislative Support} \times \left(\frac{\text{Community Engagement}}{\text{Equity in Access}} \right)$$

Assessing the impact of public policies involves the policy impact index, combining legislative support, community engagement, and equity in access.

Advocacy Effectiveness Equation:

$$\text{Advocacy Effectiveness} = \frac{\text{Public Awareness}}{\text{Policy Implementation} \times \text{Stigma Reduction}}$$

Measuring the effectiveness of advocacy includes the advocacy effectiveness equation, evaluating public awareness, policy implementation, and stigma reduction.

Equity Equation:

$$\text{Equity} = \text{Resource Allocation} \times \left(\frac{\text{Cultural Sensitivity}}{\text{Community Representation}} \right)$$

Promoting equity in mental health involves the equity equation, combining resource allocation, cultural sensitivity, and community representation.

Policy-Advocacy Symbiosis:

$$\text{Policy-Advocacy} = \frac{\text{Mental Health Legislation}}{\text{Public Support} \times \text{Collaborative Partnerships}}$$

Fostering a symbiotic relationship between policy and advocacy requires the policy-advocacy symbiosis, assessing mental health legislation, public support, and collaborative partnerships.

These symbolic equations offer a creative way to represent public policy and advocacy in community psychiatry, emphasizing factors impacting policy impact, advocacy effectiveness, equity, and the policy-advocacy symbiosis.

Chapter 10

Cultural Psychiatry

10.1 Cultural Competence in Practice

Cultural Responsiveness Index:

$$\text{Cultural Responsiveness} = \text{Cultural Awareness} \times \left(\frac{\text{Language Proficiency}}{\text{Cultural Adaptability}} \right)$$

Promoting cultural competence in practice involves the cultural responsiveness index, combining cultural awareness, language proficiency, and cultural adaptability.

Cultural Humility Equation:

$$\text{Cultural Humility} = \frac{\text{Self-Reflection}}{\text{Open-minded Communication} \times \text{Continuous Learning}}$$

Fostering cultural humility includes the cultural humility equation, evaluating self-reflection, open-minded communication, and continuous learning.

Intersectionality Harmony:

$$\text{Intersectionality} = \text{Understanding Diversity} \times \left(\frac{\text{Social Justice Advocacy}}{\text{Equitable Treatment}} \right)$$

Practicing cultural competence involves intersectionality harmony, combining understanding diversity, social justice advocacy, and equitable treatment.

Cultural Competence Quotient:

$$\text{Cultural Competence} = \frac{\text{Cultural Knowledge}}{\text{Cultural Skill Application} \times \text{Respectful Attitude}}$$

Measuring cultural competence includes the cultural competence quotient, assessing cultural knowledge, cultural skill application, and a respectful attitude.

These symbolic equations offer a creative way to represent cultural competence in practice in cultural psychiatry, emphasizing factors impacting cultural responsiveness, cultural humility, intersectionality harmony, and cultural competence.

10.2   Impact of Culture on Diagnosis

Cultural Perception Equation:

$$\text{Cultural Perception} = \text{Cultural Beliefs} \times \left(\frac{\text{Communication Styles}}{\text{Help-Seeking Norms}} \right)$$

Understanding the impact of culture on diagnosis involves the cultural perception equation, combining cultural beliefs, communication styles, and help-seeking norms.

Diagnostic Pluralism Index:

$$\text{Diagnostic Pluralism} = \frac{\text{Cultural Syndromes Recognition}}{\text{Cross-Cultural Symptom Expression} \times \text{Cultural Idioms of Distress}}$$

Assessing the diversity in diagnosis includes the diagnostic pluralism index, evaluating cultural syndromes recognition, cross-cultural symptom expression, and cultural idioms of distress.

Cultural Bias Awareness:

$$\text{Cultural Bias} = \text{Cultural Competence} \times \left(\frac{\text{Cultural Formulation Interviews}}{\text{Cultural Specificity Recognition}} \right)$$

Addressing cultural bias in diagnosis involves cultural bias awareness, combining cultural competence, cultural formulation interviews, and cultural specificity recognition.

Cultural Sensitivity Quotient:

$$\text{Cultural Sensitivity} = \frac{\text{Cultural Context Integration}}{\text{Cultural Boundaries Awareness} \times \text{Cultural Competency Training}}$$

Enhancing cultural sensitivity in diagnosis includes the cultural sensitivity quotient, assessing cultural context integration, cultural boundaries awareness, and cultural competency training.

These symbolic equations offer a creative way to represent the impact of culture on diagnosis in cultural psychiatry, emphasizing factors impacting cultural perception, diagnostic pluralism, cultural bias awareness, and cultural sensitivity.

10.3 Cross-Cultural Therapeutic Approaches

Cultural Harmony Equation:

$$\text{Cultural Harmony} = \text{Cultural Awareness} \times \left(\frac{\text{Interpersonal Flexibility}}{\text{Cultural Adaptation Strategies}} \right)$$

Fostering cultural harmony in therapeutic approaches involves the cultural harmony equation, combining cultural awareness, interpersonal flexibility, and cultural adaptation strategies.

Therapeutic Rapport Index:

$$\text{Therapeutic Rapport} = \frac{\text{Cultural Empathy}}{\text{Communication Synchrony} \times \text{Trust Building}}$$

Building rapport in cross-cultural therapeutic approaches includes the therapeutic rapport index, evaluating cultural empathy, communication synchrony, and trust-building.

Cultural Resilience Harmony:

$$\text{Cultural Resilience} = \text{Identity Affirmation} \times \left(\frac{\text{Community Support}}{\text{Trauma-Informed Interventions}} \right)$$

Promoting cultural resilience involves cultural resilience harmony, combining identity affirmation, community support, and trauma-informed interventions.

Cultural Integration Quotient:

$$\text{Cultural Integration} = \frac{\text{Cross-Cultural Psychoeducation}}{\text{Cultural Sensitivity Training} \times \text{Spiritual Inclusivity}}$$

Enhancing cultural integration in therapeutic approaches includes the cultural integration quotient, assessing cross-cultural psychoeducation, cultural sensitivity training, and spiritual inclusivity.

These symbolic equations offer a creative way to represent cross-cultural therapeutic approaches in cultural psychiatry, emphasizing factors impacting cultural harmony, therapeutic rapport, cultural resilience, and cultural integration.

10.4 Immigrant and Refugee Mental Health

Acculturation Balance Equation:

$$\text{Acculturation Balance} = \text{Cultural Retention} \times \left(\frac{\text{Adaptation Resilience}}{\text{Cultural Identity Integration}} \right)$$

Finding a balance in acculturation involves the acculturation balance equation, combining cultural retention, adaptation resilience, and cultural identity integration.

Trauma-Informed Resettlement Index:

$$\text{Trauma-Informed Resettlement} = \frac{\text{Cultural Trauma Acknowledgment}}{\text{Social Support Networks} \times \text{Community Resources Access}}$$

Navigating trauma-informed resettlement includes the trauma-informed resettlement index, evaluating cultural trauma acknowledgment, social support networks, and community resources access.

Cultural Transition Harmony:

$$\text{Cultural Transition} = \text{Cultural Navigation Skills} \times \left(\frac{\text{Language Proficiency}}{\text{Cultural Sensitivity in Healthcare}}\right)$$

Smooth cultural transitions involve cultural transition harmony, combining cultural navigation skills, language proficiency, and cultural sensitivity in healthcare.

Refugee Mental Wellbeing Quotient:

$$\text{Refugee Mental Wellbeing} = \frac{\text{Resilience Factors}}{\text{Trauma-Informed Interventions} \times \text{Social Inclusion Support}}$$

Promoting refugee mental wellbeing includes the refugee mental wellbeing quotient, assessing resilience factors, trauma-informed interventions, and social inclusion support.

These symbolic equations offer a creative way to represent immigrant and refugee mental health in cultural psychiatry, emphasizing factors impacting acculturation balance, trauma-informed resettlement, cultural transition, and refugee mental wellbeing.

10.5   Cultural Psychiatry Research

Cultural Diversity Index:

$$\text{Cultural Diversity} = \text{Ethnic Representation} \times \left(\frac{\text{Cultural Practices Study}}{\text{Language Variability}}\right)$$

Assessing cultural diversity in research involves the cultural diversity index, combining ethnic representation, cultural practices study, and language variability.

Cultural Influence Equation:

$$\text{Cultural Influence} = \frac{\text{Cultural Contextualization}}{\text{Cultural Dynamics Analysis} \times \text{Cultural Impact Assessment}}$$

Understanding the impact of culture in research includes the cultural influence equation, evaluating cultural contextualization, cultural dynamics analysis, and cultural impact assessment.

Cultural Phenomena Harmony:

$$\text{Cultural Phenomena} = \text{Cultural Belief Exploration} \times \left(\frac{\text{Cultural Phenomena Measurement}}{\text{Cultural Psychiatry Innovation}} \right)$$

Exploring cultural phenomena in research involves cultural phenomena harmony, combining cultural belief exploration, cultural phenomena measurement, and cultural psychiatry innovation.

Cultural Neuroscience Quotient:

$$\text{Cultural Neuroscience} = \frac{\text{Neurobiological Correlates Exploration}}{\text{Cultural Sensitivity in Imaging} \times \text{Cross-Cultural Neurobehavioral Studies}}$$

Advancing cultural psychiatry through neuroscience includes the cultural neuroscience quotient, assessing neurobiological correlates exploration, cultural sensitivity in imaging, and cross-cultural neurobehavioral studies.

These symbolic equations offer a creative way to represent cultural psychiatry research, emphasizing factors impacting cultural diversity, cultural influence, cultural phenomena, and cultural neuroscience.

10.6 Global Perspectives in Psychiatry

Cultural Exchange Equation:

$$\text{Cultural Exchange} = \text{Interdisciplinary Collaboration} \times \left(\frac{\text{Cross-Cultural Research}}{\text{International Partnerships}} \right)$$

Embracing global perspectives in psychiatry involves the cultural exchange equation, combining interdisciplinary collaboration, cross-cultural research, and international partnerships.

Cultural Epidemiology Index:

$$\text{Cultural Epidemiology} = \frac{\text{Global Mental Health Prevalence}}{\text{Cultural Risk Factors} \times \text{Cultural Protective Factors}}$$

Understanding mental health on a global scale includes the cultural epidemiology index, evaluating global mental health prevalence, cultural risk factors, and cultural protective factors.

Global Mental Health Equity Harmony:

$$\text{Global Mental Health Equity} = \text{Access to Treatment} \times \left(\frac{\text{Cultural Competency Policies}}{\text{Resource Allocation Equality}} \right)$$

Advancing global mental health equity involves global mental health equity harmony, combining access to treatment, cultural competency policies, and resource allocation equality.

Cultural Collaboration Quotient:

$$\text{Cultural Collaboration} = \frac{\text{Cultural Psychiatry Publications}}{\text{Multicultural Training Initiatives} \times \text{Global Mental Health Advocacy}}$$

Promoting cultural collaboration in psychiatry research includes the cultural collaboration quotient, assessing cultural psychiatry publications, multicultural training initiatives, and global mental health advocacy.

These symbolic equations offer a creative way to represent global perspectives in psychiatry, emphasizing factors impacting cultural exchange, cultural epidemiology, global mental health equity, and cultural collaboration.

Chapter 11

Emergency Psychiatry

11.1 Psychiatric Emergencies

Crisis Response Equation:

$$\text{Crisis Response} = \text{Risk Assessment} \times \left(\frac{\text{Safety Planning}}{\text{Therapeutic Alliance}} \right)$$

Addressing psychiatric emergencies involves the crisis response equation, combining risk assessment, safety planning, and therapeutic alliance.

Urgency Severity Index:

$$\text{Urgency Severity} = \frac{\text{Acute Distress Level}}{\text{Danger to Self or Others} \times \text{Access to Support}}$$

Evaluating urgency severity in emergencies includes the urgency severity index, assessing acute distress level, danger to self or others, and access to support.

Stabilization Harmony:

$$\text{Stabilization} = \text{Symptom Management} \times \left(\frac{\text{Crisis Intervention Skills}}{\text{Collaborative Decision-Making}} \right)$$

Achieving stabilization in psychiatric emergencies involves stabilization harmony, combining symptom management, crisis intervention skills, and collaborative decision-making.

Emergency Response Quotient:

$$\text{Emergency Response} = \frac{\text{Timely Intervention}}{\text{Cultural Sensitivity} \times \text{Resource Availability}}$$

Providing effective emergency response includes the emergency response quotient, assessing timely intervention, cultural sensitivity, and resource availability.

These symbolic equations offer a creative way to represent psychiatric emergencies in emergency psychiatry, emphasizing factors impacting crisis response, urgency severity, stabilization, and emergency response.

11.2   Suicide Risk Assessment

Suicidal Ideation Equation:

$$\text{Suicidal Ideation} = \text{Hopelessness} \times \left(\frac{\text{Perceived Burden}}{\text{Connectedness to Others}} \right)$$

Assessing suicidal ideation involves the suicidal ideation equation, combining hopelessness, perceived burden, and connectedness to others.

Risk Factors Index:

$$\text{Risk Factors} = \frac{\text{Psychological Pain}}{\text{Previous Suicide Attempts} \times \text{Family History of Suicide}}$$

Evaluating risk factors in suicide risk assessment includes the risk factors index, assessing psychological pain, previous suicide attempts, and family history of suicide.

Protective Factors Harmony:

$$\text{Protective Factors} = \text{Coping Skills} \times \left(\frac{\text{Access to Mental Health Resources}}{\text{Positive Life Events}} \right)$$

Considering protective factors involves protective factors harmony, combining coping skills, access to mental health resources, and positive life events.

Suicide Risk Quotient:

$$\text{Suicide Risk} = \frac{\text{Immediate Lethality}}{\text{Cultural Competence in Assessment} \times \text{Safety Planning}}$$

Evaluating suicide risk includes the suicide risk quotient, assessing immediate lethality, cultural competence in assessment, and safety planning.

These symbolic equations offer a creative way to represent suicide risk assessment in emergency psychiatry, emphasizing factors impacting suicidal ideation, risk factors, protective factors, and suicide risk.

11.3   Management of Agitation

Agitation Control Equation:

$$\text{Agitation Control} = \text{De-escalation Techniques} \times \left(\frac{\text{Environmental Modification}}{\text{Verbal Communication Strategies}} \right)$$

Managing agitation involves the agitation control equation, combining de-escalation techniques, environmental modification, and verbal communication strategies.

Crisis Stabilization Index:

$$\text{Crisis Stabilization} = \frac{\text{Anxiety Level}}{\text{Physical Restraints} \times \text{Pharmacological Intervention}}$$

Stabilizing crises in agitation management includes the crisis stabilization index, evaluating anxiety level, physical restraints, and pharmacological intervention.

Emotional Regulation Harmony:

$$\text{Emotional Regulation} = \text{Mindfulness Practices} \times \left(\frac{\text{Empathy and Validation}}{\text{Distraction Techniques}} \right)$$

Promoting emotional regulation involves emotional regulation harmony, combining mindfulness practices, empathy and validation, and distraction techniques.

Agitation Intervention Quotient:

$$\text{Agitation Intervention} = \frac{\text{Immediate Safety Measures}}{\text{Cultural Sensitivity in Intervention} \times \text{Collaborative Decision-Making}}$$

Implementing effective agitation intervention includes the agitation intervention quotient, assessing immediate safety measures, cultural sensitivity in intervention, and collaborative decision-making.

These symbolic equations offer a creative way to represent the management of agitation in emergency psychiatry, emphasizing factors impacting agitation control, crisis stabilization, emotional regulation, and agitation intervention.

11.4   Substance-Induced Psychiatric Crises

Intoxication Equation:

$$\text{Intoxication} = \text{Substance Blood Level} \times \left(\frac{\text{Clinical Symptoms}}{\text{Physiological Effects}} \right)$$

Assessing intoxication in substance-induced crises involves the intoxication equation, combining substance blood level, clinical symptoms, and physiological effects.

Withdrawal Severity Index:

$$\text{Withdrawal Severity} = \frac{\text{Duration of Substance Use}}{\text{Previous Withdrawal Episodes} \times \text{Neurobiological Vulnerability}}$$

Evaluating withdrawal severity in substance-induced crises includes the withdrawal severity index, assessing the duration of substance use, previous withdrawal episodes, and neurobiological vulnerability.

Detoxification Harmony:

$$\text{Detoxification} = \text{Medical Monitoring} \times \left(\frac{\text{Psychoeducation}}{\text{Pharmacological Support}} \right)$$

Managing detoxification in substance-induced crises involves detoxification harmony, combining medical monitoring, psychoeducation, and pharmacological support.

Substance Crisis Quotient:

$$\text{Substance Crisis} = \frac{\text{Risk of Harm to Self or Others}}{\text{Cultural Competence in Assessment} \times \text{Collaborative Treatment Planning}}$$

Navigating substance-induced psychiatric crises includes the substance crisis quotient, assessing the risk of harm to self or others, cultural competence in assessment, and collaborative treatment planning.

These symbolic equations offer a creative way to represent substance-induced psychiatric crises in emergency psychiatry, emphasizing factors impacting intoxication, withdrawal severity, detoxification, and substance crisis.

11.5   Trauma and Crisis Intervention

Trauma Resilience Equation:

$$\text{Trauma Resilience} = \text{Coping Strategies} \times \left(\frac{\text{Social Support}}{\text{Post-Traumatic Growth}} \right)$$

Addressing trauma in crisis intervention involves the trauma resilience equation, combining coping strategies, social support, and post-traumatic growth.

Crisis Debriefing Index:

$$\text{Crisis Debriefing} = \frac{\text{Immediate Crisis Response}}{\text{Emotional Processing} \times \text{Safety Planning}}$$

Debriefing in crisis intervention includes the crisis debriefing index, assessing immediate crisis response, emotional processing, and safety planning.

Empowerment Harmony:

$$\text{Empowerment} = \text{Advocacy Skills} \times \left(\frac{\text{Self-Efficacy}}{\text{Cultural Competence in Intervention}} \right)$$

Promoting empowerment in trauma and crisis intervention involves empowerment harmony, combining advocacy skills, self-efficacy, and cultural competence in intervention.

Trauma Intervention Quotient:

$$\text{Trauma Intervention} = \frac{\text{Immediate Support}}{\text{Cultural Sensitivity in Assessment} \times \text{Collaborative Decision-Making}}$$

Implementing effective trauma intervention includes the trauma intervention quotient, assessing immediate support, cultural sensitivity in assessment, and collaborative decision-making.

These symbolic equations offer a creative way to represent trauma and crisis intervention in emergency psychiatry, emphasizing factors impacting trauma resilience, crisis debriefing, empowerment, and trauma intervention.

11.6 Telepsychiatry in Emergencies

Virtual Crisis Response Equation:

$$\text{Virtual Crisis Response} = \text{Telecommunication Platforms} \times \left(\frac{\text{Remote Assessment Skills}}{\text{Technological Accessibility}} \right)$$

Engaging in virtual crisis response involves the virtual crisis response equation, combining telecommunication platforms, remote assessment skills, and technological accessibility.

Distance Crisis Stabilization Index:

$$\text{Distance Crisis Stabilization} = \frac{\text{Remote Supportive Interventions}}{\text{Digital Safety Planning} \times \text{Online Resources}}$$

Stabilizing crises through telepsychiatry includes the distance crisis stabilization index, assessing remote supportive interventions, digital safety planning, and online resources.

Tech-Mindfulness Harmony:

$$\text{Tech-Mindfulness} = \text{Virtual Mindfulness Practices} \times \left(\frac{\text{Empathy in Digital Communication}}{\text{User-Friendly Platforms}} \right)$$

Promoting tech-mindfulness in telepsychiatry involves tech-mindfulness harmony, combining virtual mindfulness practices, empathy in digital communication, and user-friendly platforms.

Telepsychiatry Effectiveness Quotient:

$$\text{Telepsychiatry Effectiveness} =$$

$$\frac{\text{Timely Virtual Intervention}}{\text{Cultural Competence in Telepsychiatry} \times \text{Collaborative Digital Decision-Making}}$$

Ensuring telepsychiatry effectiveness includes the telepsychiatry effectiveness quotient, assessing timely virtual intervention, cultural competence in telepsychiatry, and collaborative digital decision-making.

These symbolic equations offer a creative way to represent telepsychiatry in emergencies, emphasizing factors impacting virtual crisis response, distance crisis stabilization, tech-mindfulness, and telepsychiatry effectiveness.

Chapter 12

Technology in Psychiatry

12.1 Telepsychiatry and Teletherapy

Virtual Mental Wellness Equation:

$$\text{Virtual Mental Wellness} = \text{Telecommunication Platforms} \times \left(\frac{\text{Remote Assessment Skills}}{\text{User Accessibility}} \right)$$

Promoting virtual mental wellness through telepsychiatry involves the virtual mental wellness equation, combining telecommunication platforms, remote assessment skills, and user accessibility.

Distance Therapeutic Effectiveness Index:

$$\text{Distance Therapeutic Effectiveness} = \frac{\text{Remote Therapeutic Interventions}}{\text{Digital Accessibility} \times \text{Online Resources}}$$

Ensuring therapeutic effectiveness in teletherapy includes the distance therapeutic effectiveness index, assessing remote therapeutic interventions, digital accessibility, and online resources.

Tech-Enhanced Empathy Harmony:

$$\text{Tech-Enhanced Empathy} = \text{Virtual Empathy Building Exercises} \times \left(\frac{\text{Cultural Competence in Teletherapy}}{\text{User-Friendly Platforms}} \right)$$

Enhancing empathy through technology in teletherapy involves tech-enhanced empathy harmony, combining virtual empathy building exercises, cultural competence in teletherapy, and user-friendly platforms.

Telehealth Equity Quotient:

$$\text{Telehealth Equity} = \frac{\text{Accessible Virtual Intervention}}{\text{Equitable Digital Access} \times \text{Collaborative Digital Inclusivity}}$$

Ensuring telehealth equity includes the telehealth equity quotient, assessing accessible virtual intervention, equitable digital access, and collaborative digital inclusivity.

These symbolic equations offer a creative way to represent telepsychiatry and teletherapy in technology in psychiatry, emphasizing factors impacting virtual mental wellness, distance therapeutic effectiveness, tech-enhanced empathy, and telehealth equity.

12.2   Digital Mental Health Apps

App-Based Wellness Equation:

$$\text{App-Based Wellness} = \text{App Features} \times \left(\frac{\text{User Engagement}}{\text{Content Relevance}} \right)$$

Enhancing mental wellness through digital mental health apps involves the app-based wellness equation, combining app features, user engagement, and content relevance.

Virtual Therapeutic Effectiveness Index:

$$\text{Virtual Therapeutic Effectiveness} = \frac{\text{Interactive Therapeutic Modules}}{\text{User Accessibility} \times \text{In-App Resources}}$$

Ensuring therapeutic effectiveness in digital mental health apps includes the virtual therapeutic effectiveness index, assessing interactive therapeutic modules, user accessibility, and in-app resources.

Algorithmic Well-Being Harmony:

$$\text{Algorithmic Well-Being} = \text{User Data Privacy Measures} \times \left(\frac{\text{Personalized Interventions}}{\text{Algorithmic Fairness}} \right)$$

Safeguarding well-being through algorithms in mental health apps involves algorithmic well-being harmony, combining user data privacy measures, personalized interventions, and algorithmic fairness.

Mobile Mental Resilience Quotient:

$$\text{Mobile Mental Resilience} = \frac{\text{Accessible Supportive Features}}{\text{Equitable App Access} \times \text{Community Collaboration}}$$

Ensuring mobile mental resilience includes the mobile mental resilience quotient, assessing accessible supportive features, equitable app access, and community collaboration.

These symbolic equations offer a creative way to represent digital mental health apps in technology in psychiatry, emphasizing factors impacting app-based wellness, virtual therapeutic effectiveness, algorithmic well-being, and mobile mental resilience.

12.3 Artificial Intelligence in Diagnosis

AI Diagnostic Precision Formula:

$$\text{AI Diagnostic Precision} = \text{Algorithm Accuracy} \times \left(\frac{\text{Clinical Validity}}{\text{Data Diversity}} \right)$$

Leveraging artificial intelligence for diagnosis involves the AI diagnostic precision formula, combining algorithm accuracy, clinical validity, and data diversity.

Virtual Differential Diagnosis Index:

$$\text{Virtual Differential Diagnosis} = \frac{\text{Automated Symptom Analysis}}{\text{User Input} \times \text{Evidence-Based Algorithms}}$$

Ensuring a comprehensive virtual differential diagnosis through AI includes the virtual differential diagnosis index, assessing automated symptom analysis, user input, and evidence-based algorithms.

Algorithmic Therapeutic Suggestions Harmony:

$$\text{Algorithmic Therapeutic Suggestions} = \text{Personalized Treatment Algorithms} \times \left(\frac{\text{Ethical AI Practices}}{\text{Interdisciplinary Integration}} \right)$$

Providing therapeutic suggestions through AI involves algorithmic therapeutic suggestions harmony, combining personalized treatment algorithms, ethical AI practices, and interdisciplinary integration.

Neural Network Emotional Intelligence Quotient:

$$\text{Neural Network Emotional Intelligence} = \frac{\text{Emotion Recognition Accuracy}}{\text{User Feedback} \times \text{Cultural Sensitivity}}$$

Measuring emotional intelligence through AI includes the neural network emotional intelligence quotient, assessing emotion recognition accuracy, user feedback, and cultural sensitivity.

These symbolic equations offer a creative way to represent artificial intelligence in diagnosis in technology in psychiatry, emphasizing factors impacting AI diagnostic precision, virtual differential diagnosis, algorithmic therapeutic suggestions, and neural network emotional intelligence.

12.4 Virtual Reality Therapies

Immersive Healing Equation:

$$\text{Immersive Healing} = \text{Virtual Environments} \times \left(\frac{\text{Therapeutic Interactions}}{\text{User Engagement}} \right)$$

Facilitating healing through virtual reality therapies involves the immersive healing equation, combining virtual environments, therapeutic interactions, and user engagement.

Virtual Exposure Resilience Index:

$$\text{Virtual Exposure Resilience} = \frac{\text{Simulated Exposure Intensity}}{\text{User Adaptability} \times \text{In-VR Supportive Elements}}$$

Building resilience through virtual exposure in therapy includes the virtual exposure resilience index, assessing simulated exposure intensity, user adaptability, and in-VR supportive elements.

Simulation Empathy Harmony:

$$\text{Simulation Empathy} = \text{Realistic Virtual Scenarios} \times \left(\frac{\text{Cultural Sensitivity in VR Therapies}}{\text{Immersive Emotional Impact}} \right)$$

Enhancing empathy through simulation in virtual reality therapies involves simulation empathy harmony, combining realistic virtual scenarios, cultural sensitivity in VR therapies, and immersive emotional impact.

VR Therapeutic Presence Quotient:

$$\text{VR Therapeutic Presence} = \frac{\text{Immersive Therapeutic Presence}}{\text{Equitable VR Access} \times \text{Collaborative VR Integration}}$$

Ensuring therapeutic presence in virtual reality therapies includes the VR therapeutic presence quotient, assessing immersive therapeutic presence, equitable VR access, and collaborative VR integration.

These symbolic equations offer a creative way to represent virtual reality therapies in technology in psychiatry, emphasizing factors impacting immersive healing, virtual exposure resilience, simulation empathy, and VR therapeutic presence.

12.5   Ethical Considerations in Technology

Digital Ethics Equation:

$$\text{Digital Ethics} = \text{Privacy Safeguards} \times \left(\frac{\text{Algorithmic Transparency}}{\text{User Autonomy}} \right)$$

Upholding digital ethics in technology involves the digital ethics equation, combining privacy safeguards, algorithmic transparency, and user autonomy.

Equitable Tech Justice Index:

$$\text{Equitable Tech Justice} = \frac{\text{Fair Tech Distribution}}{\text{Digital Inclusivity} \times \text{Cultural Responsiveness}}$$

Ensuring tech justice with equity includes the equitable tech justice index, assessing fair tech distribution, digital inclusivity, and cultural responsiveness.

Integrity in Innovation Harmony:

$$\text{Integrity in Innovation} = \text{Ethical AI Development} \times \left(\frac{\text{User Empowerment Features}}{\text{Ethical Tech Design}} \right)$$

Harmonizing integrity in innovation involves the integrity in innovation equation, combining ethical AI development, user empowerment features, and ethical tech design.

User-Centered Consent Quotient:

$$\text{User-Centered Consent} = \frac{\text{Informed User Consent}}{\text{Transparent Data Handling} \times \text{Respectful User Control}}$$

Ensuring user-centered consent includes the user-centered consent quotient, assessing informed user consent, transparent data handling, and respectful user control.

These symbolic equations offer a creative way to represent ethical considerations in technology in psychiatry, emphasizing factors impacting digital ethics, equitable tech justice, integrity in innovation, and user-centered consent.

12.6 Future Trends

Innovation Acceleration Quotient:

$$\text{Innovation Acceleration} = \text{Emerging Technologies Integration} \times \left(\frac{\text{Interdisciplinary Collaboration}}{\text{User-Centered Design}} \right)$$

Predicting the trajectory of innovation acceleration involves the innovation acceleration quotient, combining emerging technologies integration, interdisciplinary collaboration, and user-centered design.

Neurotech Advancement Index:

$$\text{Neurotech Advancement} = \frac{\text{Neural Interface Development}}{\text{Ethical Neurotech Implementation} \times \text{Neurodiversity Considerations}}$$

Anticipating advancements in neurotechnology includes the neurotech advancement index, assessing neural interface development, ethical neurotech implementation, and neurodiversity considerations.

Psychobotics Harmony Equation:

$$\text{Psychobotics Harmony} = \text{Human-Robot Therapeutic Synergy} \times \left(\frac{\text{Emotionally Intelligent AI}}{\text{Ethical Robotics Design}} \right)$$

Exploring the harmonious integration of psychobotics involves the psychobotics harmony equation, combining human-robot therapeutic synergy, emotionally intelligent AI, and ethical robotics design.

Mind-Machine Symbiosis Quotient:

$$\text{Mind-Machine Symbiosis} = \frac{\text{Brain-Computer Interface Efficacy}}{\text{User Empowerment in Cognitive Enhancement} \times \text{Neuroethical Safeguards}}$$

Understanding the future of mind-machine symbiosis includes the mind-machine symbiosis quotient, assessing brain-computer interface efficacy, user empowerment in cognitive enhancement, and neuroethical safeguards.

These symbolic equations offer a creative way to represent future trends in technology in psychiatry, emphasizing factors impacting innovation acceleration, neurotech advancement, psychobotics harmony, and mind-machine symbiosis.

Chapter 13

Professional Development

13.1 Continuing Medical Education (CME)

CME Mastery Equation:

$$\text{CME Mastery} = \text{Active Learning Strategies} \times \left(\frac{\text{Peer Collaboration}}{\text{Self-Assessment and Reflection}} \right)$$

Achieving mastery in Continuing Medical Education involves the CME mastery equation, combining active learning strategies, peer collaboration, and self-assessment and reflection.

Knowledge Amplification Index:

$$\text{Knowledge Amplification} = \frac{\text{Up-to-Date Resources Utilization}}{\text{Interactive Learning Platforms} \times \text{Cross-Specialty Integration}}$$

Amplifying knowledge through CME includes the knowledge amplification index, assessing up-to-date resources utilization, interactive learning platforms, and cross-specialty integration.

Clinical Skills Enhancement Quotient:

$$\text{Clinical Skills Enhancement} = \text{Simulated Patient Encounters} \times \left(\frac{\text{Multimodal Instructional Approaches}}{\text{Application in Real Patient Care}} \right)$$

Enhancing clinical skills through CME involves the clinical skills enhancement quotient, combining simulated patient encounters, multimodal instructional approaches, and application in real patient care.

Ethical Decision-making Index:

$$\text{Ethical Decision-making} = \frac{\text{Case-based Ethics Training}}{\text{Professionalism Reinforcement} \times \text{Cultural Competence Integration}}$$

Fostering ethical decision-making in CME includes the ethical decision-making index, assessing case-based ethics training, professionalism reinforcement, and cultural competence integration.

These symbolic equations offer a creative way to represent continuing medical education (CME), emphasizing factors impacting CME mastery, knowledge amplification, clinical skills enhancement, and ethical decision-making.

13.2   Board Certification and Licensing

Certification Success Formula:

$$\text{Certification Success} = \text{Comprehensive Exam Preparation} \times \left(\frac{\text{Clinical Proficiency}}{\text{Evidence-Based Knowledge}} \right)$$

Attaining success in board certification involves the certification success formula, combining comprehensive exam preparation, clinical proficiency, and evidence-based knowledge.

Licensing Resilience Equation:

$$\text{Licensing Resilience} = \frac{\text{Regulatory Compliance}}{\text{Continuous Professional Development} \times \text{Ethical Practice}}$$

Fostering resilience in licensing involves the licensing resilience equation, assessing regulatory compliance, continuous professional development, and ethical practice.

Competency Validation Index:

$$\text{Competency Validation} = \text{Performance Assessments} \times \left(\frac{\text{Peer Evaluations}}{\text{Ongoing Learning Plans}} \right)$$

Validating competency in board certification and licensing includes the competency validation index, combining performance assessments, peer evaluations, and ongoing learning plans.

Moral Fitness Quotient:

$$\text{Moral Fitness} = \frac{\text{Ethics Education}}{\text{Professional Integrity} \times \text{Patient Advocacy}}$$

Ensuring moral fitness in professional development involves the moral fitness quotient, assessing ethics education, professional integrity, and patient advocacy.

These symbolic equations offer a creative way to represent board certification and licensing, emphasizing factors impacting certification success, licensing resilience, competency validation, and moral fitness.

13.3 Career Pathways in Psychiatry

Career Flourishing Equation:

$$\text{Career Flourishing} = \text{Clinical Expertise} \times \left(\frac{\text{Research Impact}}{\text{Community Engagement}} \right)$$

Navigating career pathways in psychiatry involves the career flourishing equation, combining clinical expertise, research impact, and community engagement.

Leadership Prowess Index:

$$\text{Leadership Prowess} = \frac{\text{Strategic Decision-Making}}{\text{Team Collaboration} \times \text{Innovation Adoption}}$$

Cultivating leadership prowess in psychiatry includes the leadership prowess index, assessing strategic decision-making, team collaboration, and innovation adoption.

Education Empowerment Quotient:

$$\text{Education Empowerment} = \text{Mentorship Quality} \times \left(\frac{\text{Teaching Excellence}}{\text{Lifelong Learning Commitment}} \right)$$

Empowering education in psychiatry involves the education empowerment quotient, combining mentorship quality, teaching excellence, and lifelong learning commitment.

Balance Harmony Factor:

$$\text{Balance Harmony} = \frac{\text{Work-Life Integration}}{\text{Wellness Advocacy} \times \text{Resilience Cultivation}}$$

Achieving balance in career pathways includes the balance harmony factor, assessing work-life integration, wellness advocacy, and resilience cultivation.

These symbolic equations offer a creative way to represent career pathways in psychiatry, emphasizing factors impacting career flourishing, leadership prowess, education empowerment, and balance harmony.

13.4 Mentorship in Psychiatry

Mentorship Impact Equation:

$$\text{Mentorship Impact} = \text{Guidance Quality} \times \left(\frac{\text{Career Advancement Support}}{\text{Research Collaboration}} \right)$$

Embarking on mentorship in psychiatry involves the mentorship impact equation, combining guidance quality, career advancement support, and research collaboration.

Empowerment Matrix:

$$\text{Empowerment} = \frac{\text{Skills Transfer}}{\text{Networking Opportunities} \times \text{Diversity Inclusion}}$$

Fostering empowerment in mentorship includes the empowerment matrix, assessing skills transfer, networking opportunities, and diversity inclusion.

Wisdom Transfer Index:

$$\text{Wisdom Transfer} = \text{Experience Sharing} \times \left(\frac{\text{Life Balance Insights}}{\text{Professional Growth Reflection}}\right)$$

Facilitating wisdom transfer in psychiatry involves the wisdom transfer index, combining experience sharing, life balance insights, and professional growth reflection.

Cultural Alchemy Quotient:

$$\text{Cultural Alchemy} = \frac{\text{Cultural Competence Boost}}{\text{Inclusivity Promotion} \times \text{Collaborative Learning}}$$

Promoting cultural alchemy in mentorship includes the cultural alchemy quotient, assessing cultural competence boost, inclusivity promotion, and collaborative learning.

These symbolic equations offer a creative way to represent mentorship in psychiatry, emphasizing factors impacting mentorship impact, empowerment, wisdom transfer, and cultural alchemy.

13.5   Professional Organizations

Membership Equation:

$$\text{Membership} = \text{Networking Opportunities} \times \left(\frac{\text{Continuing Education Access}}{\text{Leadership Development Programs}}\right)$$

Engaging with professional organizations in psychiatry involves the membership equation, combining networking opportunities, access to continuing education, and participation in leadership development programs.

Collaboration Index:

$$\text{Collaboration} = \frac{\text{Interdisciplinary Connections}}{\text{Research Collaborations} \times \text{Advocacy Involvement}}$$

Fostering collaboration within professional organizations includes the collaboration index, assessing interdisciplinary connections, research collaborations, and advocacy involvement.

Innovation Quotient:

$$\text{Innovation} = \text{Technology Adoption} \times \left(\frac{\text{Best Practices Sharing}}{\text{Mentorship Initiatives}}\right)$$

Driving innovation in professional organizations involves the innovation quotient, combining technology adoption, sharing best practices, and mentorship initiatives.

Impact Amplification Factor:

$$\text{Impact Amplification} = \frac{\text{Community Outreach}}{\text{Policy Influence} \times \text{Global Initiatives}}$$

Maximizing impact within professional organizations includes the impact amplification factor, assessing community outreach, policy influence, and global initiatives.

These symbolic equations offer a creative way to represent professional organizations in psychiatry, emphasizing factors impacting membership, collaboration, innovation, and impact amplification.

13.6 Balancing Work and Well-Being

Well-Being Equation:

$$\text{Well-Being} = \text{Work-Life Balance} \times \left(\frac{\text{Physical Health}}{\text{Mental Wellness}} \right)$$

Achieving well-being while balancing work involves the well-being equation, combining work-life balance with considerations for physical health and mental wellness.

Energy Renewal Formula:

$$\text{Energy Renewal} = \frac{\text{Restorative Sleep}}{\text{Stress Resilience} \times \text{Recreational Activities}}$$

Maintaining energy levels includes the energy renewal formula, assessing the impact of restorative sleep, stress resilience, and engaging in recreational activities.

Time Management Index:

$$\text{Time Management} = \text{Efficiency} \times \left(\frac{\text{Personal Time Allocation}}{\text{Professional Commitments}} \right)$$

Effective time management in work and well-being involves the time management index, combining efficiency with considerations for personal time allocation and professional commitments.

Mindfulness Quotient:

$$\text{Mindfulness} = \frac{\text{Present-Moment Awareness}}{\text{Work-related Distractions} \times \text{Mind-Body Practices}}$$

Cultivating mindfulness includes the mindfulness quotient, assessing present-moment awareness, managing work-related distractions, and incorporating mind-body practices.

These symbolic equations offer a creative way to represent balancing work and well-being in psychiatry, emphasizing factors impacting well-being, energy renewal, time management, and mindfulness.

Chapter 14

Research in Psychiatry

14.1 Research Methodologies

Scientific Inquiry Formula:

$$\text{Scientific Inquiry} = \text{Curiosity} \times \left(\frac{\text{Hypothesis Formation}}{\text{Data Collection}} \right)$$

Embarking on scientific inquiry involves the scientific inquiry formula, combining curiosity with the process of hypothesis formation and data collection.

Statistical Significance Index:

$$\text{Statistical Significance} = \frac{\text{Effect Size}}{\text{Sample Variability} \times \text{Research Design Rigor}}$$

Assessing statistical significance includes the statistical significance index, evaluating the effect size in relation to sample variability and the rigor of the research design.

Ethical Research Quotient:

$$\text{Ethical Research} = \frac{\text{Informed Consent}}{\text{Confidentiality Assurance} \times \text{Participant Well-being}}$$

Conducting ethical research involves the ethical research quotient, emphasizing informed consent, confidentiality assurance, and ensuring participant well-being.

Innovation Factor:

$$\text{Innovation} = \text{Creative Methodologies} \times \left(\frac{\text{Technology Integration}}{\text{Cross-Disciplinary Collaboration}} \right)$$

Fostering innovation in research includes the innovation factor, incorporating creative methodologies, integrating technology, and promoting cross-disciplinary collaboration.

These symbolic equations offer a creative way to represent research methodologies in psychiatry, emphasizing curiosity, hypothesis formation, data collection, statistical significance, ethical considerations, and innovation.

14.2   Clinical Trials Symphony

In the symphony of clinical trials, researchers conduct an orchestrated exploration of therapeutic melodies. The randomized controlled trials (RCTs) serve as the conductor's baton, guiding the way to evidence-based practices in psychiatry.

14.2.1   Randomization Ballet

The randomization ballet begins, as participants dance between the experimental and control arms. Like a choreographed sequence, random assignment ensures unbiased distribution, minimizing confounding factors and enhancing the internal validity of the trial.

14.2.2   Placebo Effect Waltz

Amidst the waltz of placebo effects, researchers carefully consider the psychological impact of inert interventions. The placebo response, akin to a dance partner, underscores the importance of blinding and controls, teasing out the true efficacy of the tested interventions.

14.2.3   Double-Blind Pas de Deux

In the pas de deux of double-blind methodology, both participants and investigators twirl in uncertainty. Neither knowing who receives the active treatment or placebo, this dance safeguards against biases, contributing to the robustness of the trial's findings.

14.2.4   Statistical Tango

The statistical tango commences as data take center stage. Through intricate calculations and statistical tests, researchers evaluate the significance of findings, determining whether the observed effects are more than mere chance, adding a rhythm of precision to the clinical trial composition.

14.2.5   Longitudinal Waltz

In the longitudinal waltz, researchers follow participants over time, capturing the evolving narrative of treatment outcomes. This dance unravels the nuances of sustainability and long-term impacts, enriching the clinical understanding of interventions beyond immediate effects.

14.2.6   Adverse Events Breakdance

The breakdance of adverse events unfolds as researchers monitor for unexpected twists and turns. This vigilant choreography ensures participant safety, revealing any side effects or complications that may arise during the trial, guiding ethical practice.

14.2.7   Publication Quadrille

As the clinical trial performance concludes, the publication quadrille takes center stage. Researchers disseminate findings through peer-reviewed journals, sharing insights and contributing to the collective knowledge of psychiatric interventions.

14.2.8   Meta-Analysis Ballet

The meta-analysis ballet brings together multiple clinical trials in a grand finale. Research synthesizers perform a coordinated routine, combining results to unveil broader patterns, strengths, and limitations, enriching the landscape of evidence-based psychiatry.

These vivid metaphors encapsulate the essence of clinical trials in psychiatry, using dance and movement as analogies to convey the intricacies of randomization, placebo effects, double-blind methodology, statistical analysis, longitudinal studies, adverse event monitoring, publication processes, and meta-analytical synthesis.

14.3   Neuroscience Ballet in Psychiatry

In the captivating ballet of neuroscience and psychiatry, the intricate dance between brain function and mental health takes center stage. Let's embark on this choreographed journey, where neurons pirouette through emotions, and neurotransmitters perform a delicate pas de deux.

14.3.1   Neurotransmitter Waltz

The neurotransmitter waltz begins with serotonin, dopamine, and norepinephrine gracefully gliding across synapses. Their elegant movements influence mood, motivation, and pleasure, orchestrating a harmonious dance that is both beautiful and complex.

14.3.2   Synaptic Pas de Deux

In the synaptic pas de deux, neurons exchange information through synapses, forming the foundation of cognitive processes. The pre-synaptic axon and post-synaptic dendrite engage in a graceful interplay, transmitting signals in a choreographed sequence that underlies thoughts and emotions.

14.3.3   Neuroplasticity Ballet

The neuroplasticity ballet unfolds as the brain's adaptability takes the spotlight. Neurons engage in a dynamic performance, forming new connections and pathways in response to experiences. This ballet highlights the brain's remarkable ability to reorganize and recover.

14.3.4   Brain Imaging Symphony

The brain imaging symphony commences, with fMRI, PET, and EEG instruments harmonizing to visualize the brain's activity. Through these instruments, researchers observe the cerebral movements, unveiling the secrets of psychiatric disorders and contributing to diagnostic precision.

14.3.5   Genetic Variations Minuet

In the genetic variations minuet, the intricate steps of DNA dance on the stage of psychiatric research. Researchers uncover the subtle minuet of genetic influences, exploring how variations contribute to susceptibility or resilience in mental health disorders.

14.3.6   Neurocircuitry Rhapsody

The neurocircuitry rhapsody unfolds as researchers map the intricate pathways within the brain. This composition reveals the symphony of circuits governing mood, cognition, and behavior, providing insights into potential targets for psychiatric interventions.

14.3.7 Neuroinflammation Tango

The neuroinflammation tango takes center stage, exploring the connection between immune responses and psychiatric conditions. In this dance, researchers investigate how inflammation may contribute to the development and progression of disorders, offering new avenues for therapeutic exploration.

14.3.8 Neurochemical Equations

Amidst this ballet, neurochemical equations emerge. Consider serotonin modulation represented by the equation:

$$\text{Serotonin(5-HT)} \xleftrightarrow{\text{Enzymes}} \text{5-Hydroxyindoleacetic Acid(5-HIAA)} + \text{Metabolites}$$

Such equations depict the delicate balance of neurotransmitter dynamics, unveiling the biochemical poetry that shapes mental health.

This neuroscience ballet in psychiatry showcases the elegance and complexity of the brain's dance, intertwining molecular intricacies, neural pathways, and genetic influences into a mesmerizing performance.

14.4 Genetics Waltz in Psychiatry

In the grand ballroom of psychiatric research, the Genetics Waltz takes center stage, unraveling the intricate dance between genetic factors and mental health. Let's join this captivating performance, where the choreography of DNA dictates the rhythm of psychiatric conditions.

14.4.1 Genetic Variation Minuet

The Genetic Variation Minuet unfolds as researchers explore the subtle steps of DNA sequences. The dance of nucleotides, represented by the equation:

$$A \xleftrightarrow{\text{Genetic Variation}} T \quad \text{and} \quad C \xleftrightarrow{\text{Genetic Variation}} G$$

reveals the delicate minuet of genetic variations, influencing susceptibility or resilience to psychiatric disorders.

14.4.2   Heritability Tango

In the Heritability Tango, researchers examine the heritability of mental health conditions. The equation:

$$\text{Heritability} = \frac{\text{Genetic Variance}}{\text{Total Variance}}$$

quantifies the contribution of genetic factors, guiding our understanding of the interplay between genes and the environment in psychiatric outcomes.

14.4.3   Polygenic Score Symphony

The Polygenic Score Symphony commences, harmonizing the influence of multiple genes on psychiatric risk. This multifaceted composition, portrayed by the equation:

$$\text{Polygenic Score} = \sum_{i=1}^{n} \beta_i \times \text{Genotype}_i$$

reveals the cumulative impact of various genetic markers, orchestrating a complex melody in the realm of psychiatric genetics.

14.4.4   Genome-Wide Association Minuet

The Genome-Wide Association Minuet steps into the spotlight, exploring associations between genetic markers and psychiatric disorders. This dance, depicted by equations such as:

$$\text{GWAS} \xleftrightarrow{\text{Identify}} \text{Risk Loci}$$

guides researchers in uncovering specific genetic regions linked to mental health susceptibility.

14.4.5   Epigenetic Rhapsody

The Epigenetic Rhapsody showcases the dynamic interplay between genes and the environment. Epigenetic modifications, represented by equations like:

$$\text{Methylation} \xleftrightarrow{\text{Environmental Influence}} \text{Gene Expression}$$

reveal how environmental factors influence the activation or silencing of specific genes, adding nuanced layers to the genetics waltz.

This genetics waltz in psychiatry unfolds the complex and nuanced relationship between our genetic makeup and mental well-being, illuminating the intricate steps of this captivating dance.

14.5 Translational Psychiatry Ballet

Enter the ethereal realm of Translational Psychiatry Ballet, where the delicate pas de deux between laboratory findings and clinical applications takes center stage. Join us in this graceful dance as we bridge the gap between bench and bedside.

14.5.1 Lab Discoveries Waltz

In the Lab Discoveries Waltz, researchers twirl through the intricacies of experimental findings. The dance is choreographed with equations such as:

$$\text{Lab Discoveries} \xleftrightarrow{\text{Experimental Research}} \text{Biological Insights}$$

where molecular and cellular revelations pirouette into a deeper understanding of psychiatric mechanisms.

14.5.2 Animal Model Tango

The Animal Model Tango unfolds as researchers and their furry partners traverse the dance floor. The equation:

$$\text{Animal Models} \xleftrightarrow{\text{Behavioral Correlation}} \text{Human Relevance}$$

guides the elegant movements, ensuring that insights gained from animal studies gracefully mirror human psychiatric conditions.

14.5.3 Clinical Application Minuet

The Clinical Application Minuet commences as lab findings delicately waltz into the realm of patient care. This harmonious dance is illustrated by equations such as:

$$\text{Lab Discoveries} \xleftrightarrow{\text{Clinical Trials}} \text{Treatment Innovations}$$

allowing research to seamlessly transition from the laboratory to real-world therapeutic interventions.

14.5.4   Neuroimaging Ballet

The Neuroimaging Ballet takes the stage, incorporating visual poetry to understand the brain's dance in psychiatric disorders. The equation:

$$\text{Neuroimaging} \xleftrightarrow{\text{Brain Activity Patterns}} \text{Psychopathology}$$

unveils the choreography of neural patterns, offering a mesmerizing glimpse into the intricacies of mental health.

14.5.5   Precision Medicine Waltz

The grand finale, the Precision Medicine Waltz, orchestrates personalized treatments based on individual differences. Equations like:

$$\text{Genetic Profiles} \xleftrightarrow{\text{Treatment Response}} \text{Tailored Interventions}$$

guide this closing performance, promising a future where psychiatric care is finely tuned to each unique individual.

The Translational Psychiatry Ballet elegantly unites scientific discovery with practical applications, seamlessly bringing breakthroughs from the lab to the lives of those touched by mental health challenges.

14.6   Ethical Duet in Psychiatry Research

Embark on a journey through the moral tapestry of psychiatric research, where the delicate Ethical Duet guides every step towards scientific progress with unwavering integrity.

14.6.1   Informed Consent Waltz

In the Informed Consent Waltz, the dance partners, researchers, and participants move in synchrony. The equation:

$$\text{Informed Consent} \xleftrightarrow{\text{Participant Autonomy}} \text{Research Integrity}$$

encapsulates the respectful exchange, ensuring that participants willingly join the dance, fully aware of their role in advancing knowledge.

14.6.2   Confidentiality Foxtrot

The Confidentiality Foxtrot sees researchers and data confidentiality twirl gracefully. The equation:

$$\text{Confidentiality Assurance} \xleftrightarrow{\text{Data Security}} \text{Participant Trust}$$

forms the core of this dance, safeguarding the privacy of those who contribute to the research endeavors.

14.6.3   Equitable Access Tango

In the Equitable Access Tango, researchers and communities engage in a synchronized effort. The equation:

$$\text{Research Benefits} \xleftrightarrow{\text{Equitable Distribution}} \text{Community Well-being}$$

ensures that the fruits of research benefit all, fostering a harmonious relationship between the scientific community and the broader society.

14.6.4   Research Integrity Rumba

The Research Integrity Rumba brings a spirited dance between ethical conduct and scientific rigor. The equation:

$$\text{Research Ethics} \xleftrightarrow{\text{Scientific Validity}} \text{Public Trust}$$

defines the choreography, emphasizing that ethical standards are the foundation upon which trustworthy and impactful research stands.

14.6.5   Global Collaboration Ballet

The Global Collaboration Ballet takes center stage, promoting a dance of cultural sensitivity and international cooperation. The equation:

$$\text{Cultural Awareness} \xleftrightarrow{\text{International Collaboration}} \text{Global Progress}$$

illustrates the interconnectedness of diverse perspectives, enriching the global research landscape.

The Ethical Duet in Psychiatry Research ensures that every pirouette of progress is guided by principles that honor the dignity of participants, uphold the trust of communities, and advance knowledge with the utmost ethical standards.

Chapter 15

Quality Improvement in Psychiatry

15.1 Measuring Triumphs: Psychiatry's Quality Symphony

Embark on a melodic exploration of Outcome Measurement, where the orchestra of quality improvement plays harmoniously to assess the crescendo of psychiatric interventions.

15.1.1 Symphony of Outcome Measures

In the Symphony of Outcome Measures, different instruments, representing diverse metrics, join together. The equation:

$$\text{Clinical Outcomes} \xleftrightarrow{\text{Patient Functionality}} \text{Treatment Efficacy}$$

orchestrates a beautiful harmony, ensuring that clinical interventions resonate positively with the functional well-being of the patients.

15.1.2 Harmonic Feedback Loop

The Harmonic Feedback Loop encapsulates the continuous improvement process. The equation:

$$\text{Outcome Assessment} \xleftrightarrow{\text{Feedback Integration}} \text{Quality Refinement}$$

paves the way for a cyclical process, where feedback becomes the compass guiding refinements in the quality of psychiatric care.

15.1.3   Resonance of Patient Satisfaction

The Resonance of Patient Satisfaction echoes through the treatment landscape. The equation:

$$\text{Patient Feedback} \xleftrightarrow{\text{Quality of Care}} \text{Therapeutic Alliance}$$

establishes a bond between the care provided and the satisfaction experienced by patients, ensuring a resonant therapeutic alliance.

15.1.4   Balanced Scorecard Ballet

In the Balanced Scorecard Ballet, the dance of diverse metrics takes center stage. The equation:

$$\text{Clinical Indicators} \xleftrightarrow{\text{Operational Metrics}} \text{Quality Assessment}$$

offers a balletic display of balance, incorporating clinical indicators and operational metrics for a comprehensive quality assessment.

15.1.5   Continuous Improvement Waltz

The Continuous Improvement Waltz involves a rhythmic dance towards excellence. The equation:

$$\text{Quality Assessment} \xleftrightarrow{\text{Process Refinement}} \text{Enhanced Outcomes}$$

guides the dance, emphasizing that continuous refinement of processes is key to achieving enhanced psychiatric outcomes.

In the grand symphony of Outcome Measurement, psychiatry strives to fine-tune its practices, ensuring that each note played contributes to the overall harmony of quality improvement.

15.2   Guardians of Serenity: Patient Safety in Psychiatry

Embark on a journey through the bastions of Patient Safety in Psychiatry, guarded by vigilant equations ensuring a fortress against potential risks.

15.2.1 Sentinels of Vigilance

The Sentinels of Vigilance stand guard, symbolizing the equation:

$$\text{Risk Assessment} \xleftrightarrow{\text{Continuous Monitoring}} \text{Patient Safety}$$

This equation signifies the unwavering vigilance needed through risk assessments and continuous monitoring to safeguard the sanctuary of patient safety.

15.2.2 Safety Pharmacology Shield

The Safety Pharmacology Shield, represented by the equation:

$$\text{Pharmacological Intervention} \xleftrightarrow{\text{Adverse Effects Monitoring}} \text{Risk Mitigation}$$

acts as a protective barrier, ensuring that pharmacological interventions are coupled with vigilant monitoring to promptly mitigate any potential adverse effects.

15.2.3 Adaptive Risk Management

In the Adaptive Risk Management dance, the equation:

$$\text{Dynamic Risk Assessment} \xleftrightarrow{\text{Real-time Adjustments}} \text{Enhanced Safety}$$

guides the fluid dance of adjusting strategies in real-time, enhancing the safety protocols through dynamic risk assessment.

15.2.4 Resilience Equation

The Resilience Equation, expressed as:

$$\text{Training and Preparedness} \xleftrightarrow{\text{Crisis Response}} \text{Psychiatric Emergency Resilience}$$

embodies the essence of resilience, where training and preparedness harmonize to fortify the psychiatric domain against unforeseen crises.

15.2.5   Safety Culture Formula

The Safety Culture Formula encapsulates the equation:

$$\text{Open Communication} \xleftrightarrow{\text{Organizational Support}} \text{Patient Safety Culture}$$

cultivating an environment where open communication, supported by the organization, fosters a robust patient safety culture.

In the realm of Patient Safety in Psychiatry, these equations stand as guardians, ensuring that the fortress remains impenetrable against potential threats, fostering an environment of serenity and healing.

15.3   Harmony of Progress: Continuous Quality Improvement in Psychiatry

Embark on a journey through the symphony of Continuous Quality Improvement in Psychiatry, guided by the mathematical harmonies that propel progress.

15.3.1   Cycle of Perpetual Enhancement

The Cycle of Perpetual Enhancement is an equation that governs the process:

$$\text{Assessment} \xleftrightarrow{\text{Feedback Loops}} \text{Continuous Improvement}$$

This cycle illustrates the constant feedback loops that drive the perpetual enhancement of psychiatric practices, ensuring a dynamic and responsive system.

15.3.2   Innovative Intervention Formula

The Innovative Intervention Formula is expressed as:

$$\text{Novel Strategies} \xleftrightarrow{\text{Adaptive Implementation}} \text{Quality Leap}$$

Here, novel strategies, through adaptive implementation, become the driving force for a quantum leap in the quality of psychiatric interventions.

15.3.3 Efficiency Optimization Equation

The Efficiency Optimization Equation is captured by:

$$\text{Resource Allocation} \xleftrightarrow{\text{Process Streamlining}} \text{Enhanced Efficiency}$$

This equation signifies the synergy between judicious resource allocation and streamlined processes, leading to enhanced efficiency in psychiatric services.

15.3.4 Outcome Optimization Symphony

The Outcome Optimization Symphony orchestrates the equation:

$$\text{Data Analysis} \xleftrightarrow{\text{Evidence-Based Adjustments}} \text{Optimized Outcomes}$$

This symphony ensures that meticulous data analysis, coupled with evidence-based adjustments, harmonizes to create optimized outcomes for psychiatric care.

15.3.5 Culture of Continuous Learning

In the Culture of Continuous Learning, the equation unfolds as:

$$\text{Education and Training} \xleftrightarrow{\text{Iterative Refinement}} \text{Learning Organization}$$

This equation underscores the importance of education and training, iteratively refined, to foster a culture of continuous learning within psychiatric institutions.

In the realm of Continuous Quality Improvement, these mathematical harmonies compose the symphony of progress, guiding psychiatry towards a horizon of perpetual enhancement.

15.4 Peer Review Precision in Psychiatry

Embark on a journey through the precision of Peer Review in Psychiatry, guided by mathematical insights and equations that illuminate the path to excellence.

15.4.1 Evaluative Dynamics Formula

The Evaluative Dynamics Formula encapsulates the essence:

$$\text{Peer Evaluations} \xleftrightarrow{\text{Constructive Feedback}} \text{Refined Practices}$$

This formula symbolizes the reciprocal relationship between peer evaluations and constructive feedback, culminating in the refinement of psychiatric practices.

15.4.2 Performance Enhancement Equation

The Performance Enhancement Equation is expressed as:

$$\text{Quality Metrics} \xleftrightarrow{\text{Collaborative Assessment}} \text{Enhanced Performance}$$

In this equation, quality metrics and collaborative assessment synergize to propel enhanced performance in psychiatric care.

15.4.3 Error Minimization Algorithm

The Error Minimization Algorithm governs the equation:

$$\text{Identified Errors} \xleftrightarrow{\text{Iterative Correction}} \text{Minimized Errors}$$

This algorithm highlights the iterative process of identifying errors and implementing corrections to achieve the minimized occurrence of errors in psychiatric procedures.

15.4.4 Feedback Loop Harmony

Feedback Loop Harmony is illustrated by:

$$\text{Peer Review} \xleftrightarrow{\text{Continuous Loop}} \text{Continuous Improvement}$$

In this harmonic equation, the peer review process establishes a continuous loop, fostering an environment of perpetual improvement in psychiatric methodologies.

15.4.5 Validation Symphony

The Validation Symphony orchestrates the equation:

$$\text{Peer Recognition} \xleftrightarrow{\text{Validation Mechanisms}} \text{Professional Excellence}$$

This symphony emphasizes how peer recognition, through validation mechanisms, contributes to the attainment of professional excellence in the field of psychiatry.

Peer Review in Psychiatry, guided by these mathematical formulations, emerges as a precision instrument, finely tuning the landscape of psychiatric practices towards unparalleled excellence.

15.5 Risk Management Resilience in Psychiatry

Dive into the world of Risk Management in Psychiatry, navigating its intricacies with the aid of mathematical formulations and equations that bring clarity and precision.

15.5.1 Risk Mitigation Equation

The Risk Mitigation Equation is articulated as:

$$\text{Risk Identification} \xleftrightarrow{\text{Proactive Measures}} \text{Mitigated Risks}$$

In this equation, the proactive identification of risks interlaces with strategic measures, resulting in the effective mitigation of potential risks in psychiatric contexts.

15.5.2 Safety Index Formula

The Safety Index Formula encapsulates the relationship:

$$\text{Safety Protocols} \xleftrightarrow{\text{Implementation Efficiency}} \text{Safety Index}$$

Efficient implementation of safety protocols correlates directly with the establishment of a robust Safety Index, ensuring a secure environment within psychiatric practices.

15.5.3   Crisis Preparedness Algorithm

The Crisis Preparedness Algorithm is represented by:

$$\text{Emergency Planning} \xleftrightarrow{\text{Resource Allocation}} \text{Crisis Readiness}$$

This algorithm elucidates how meticulous emergency planning and optimal resource allocation synergize to foster a state of constant readiness for potential crises in psychiatric settings.

15.5.4   Vulnerability Quotient Dynamics

The Vulnerability Quotient Dynamics equation unfolds as:

$$\text{Risk Factors} \xleftrightarrow{\text{Adaptive Strategies}} \text{Reduced Vulnerability}$$

By adapting strategic measures in response to identified risk factors, the vulnerability quotient is systematically reduced, fortifying psychiatric practices against potential vulnerabilities.

15.5.5   Resilience Amplification

The Resilience Amplification equation is expressed as:

$$\text{Resilience Strategies} \xleftrightarrow{\text{Continuous Refinement}} \text{Amplified Resilience}$$

Continuous refinement of resilience strategies amplifies the overall resilience of psychiatric practices, ensuring robust responses to unforeseen challenges.

Risk Management in Psychiatry, as unveiled through these mathematical expressions, emerges as a fortress of resilience, fortified by strategic equations to navigate uncertainties with precision.

15.6   Optimizing Best Practices in Psychiatry

Embark on the journey of optimizing best practices in Psychiatry, where efficiency meets precision through mathematical formulations and equations.

15.6.1 Best Practices Equation

The Best Practices Equation is articulated as:

$$\text{Clinical Protocols} \xleftrightarrow{\text{Efficiency Metrics}} \text{Optimized Practices}$$

Efficiency metrics intricately link with clinical protocols, resulting in the optimization of psychiatric practices, where streamlined processes enhance overall effectiveness.

15.6.2 Quality Index Formula

The Quality Index Formula encapsulates the relationship:

$$\text{Adherence to Standards} \xleftrightarrow{\text{Process Improvement}} \text{Quality Index}$$

Strategic process improvements correlate directly with the adherence to established standards, contributing to the augmentation of the Quality Index in psychiatric care.

15.6.3 Patient Outcomes Algorithm

The Patient Outcomes Algorithm is represented by:

$$\text{Evidence-Based Interventions} \xleftrightarrow{\text{Outcome Evaluation}} \text{Enhanced Patient Outcomes}$$

This algorithm illustrates how the rigorous evaluation of outcomes, coupled with evidence-based interventions, leads to a consistent enhancement of patient outcomes in psychiatric settings.

15.6.4 Efficiency Quotient Dynamics

The Efficiency Quotient Dynamics equation unfolds as:

$$\text{Resource Allocation} \xleftrightarrow{\text{Workflow Optimization}} \text{Enhanced Efficiency}$$

Optimal allocation of resources, combined with streamlined workflow optimization, systematically enhances the overall efficiency quotient, ensuring seamless operations in psychiatric practices.

15.6.5   Continuous Improvement

The Continuous Improvement equation is expressed as:

$$\text{Feedback Integration} \xleftrightarrow{\text{Iterative Refinement}} \text{Continuous Enhancement}$$

By iteratively refining practices based on integrated feedback, continuous improvement becomes the cornerstone of psychiatric care, fostering a culture of perpetual enhancement.

Optimizing best practices in Psychiatry, as revealed through these mathematical expressions, transforms the landscape into a realm of precision and efficacy.